DYING AT HOME
WITH CANCER

DYING AT HOME
WITH CANCER

By

PATRICIA H. KENNEDY, Ph.D.

Arizona State University
Tempe, Arizona

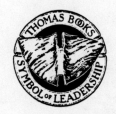

CHARLES C THOMAS • PUBLISHER
Springfield • Illinois • U.S.A.

Published and Distributed Throughout the World by
CHARLES C THOMAS • PUBLISHER
2600 South First Street
Springfield, Illinois 62717, U.S.A.

© *1982 by* CHARLES C THOMAS • PUBLISHER

ISBN 0-398-04628-X

Library of Congress Catalog Card Number: 81-14563

Printed in the United States of America
I-R.X-1

Library of Congress Cataloging in Publication Data

Kennedy, Patricia H.
    Dying at home with cancer.

    Includes index.
    1. Cancer--Patients--Home care. 2. Terminal care.
3. Right to die. 4. Death. I. Title. [DNLM: 1. Termi-
nal care--Methods. 2. Home nursing. 3. Neoplasms--
Nursing. 4. Attitude to death. WY 200 K36d]
RC262.K394   362.1'96994   81-14563
ISBN 0-398-04628-X   AACR2

To the memory of my father, William R. Kennedy

PREFACE

THIS book proposes an alternative to hospital care for terminal patients at the end of their battle with cancer. Before this point it is assumed that the patient was under the care of a physician, preferably a cancer specialist called oncologist, to make sure all measures were taken with surgery and chemotherapy to slow down the progress of the tumor. The techniques explained in this book begin when hope is given up for prolonging life any further. Methods for making the final phase of life successful and comfortable are described. They cover physical and emotional care, legal considerations, psychological aspects of death from cancer, and coping techniques for helping the patient, family members, and friends during the last stages of the dying process. The book is intended to help families care for a terminal cancer patient at home, so the advice given on topics such as how to give shots and understand medication dosages is practical in nature.

A cancer patient becomes all too familiar with hospitals. Once a diagnosis of metastatic cancer is made, the hospital becomes the scene for attempts at stopping the progress of the cancer. There the patient undergoes surgery to extract the cancer, radiation to burn it out, or chemotherapy to poison it. Finally, if cancer spreads after attempts to irradicate it, the hospital becomes the holding station for patients in their last bout with cancer.

It is the final use of the hospital that is questioned. It is legitimate to routinely hospitalize patients for whom there is no cure? Does a cancer patient have an alternative to dying in a hospital? If a person had a choice about where to spend the last moments of his life, would he choose being in a hospital surrounded by strangers or would he prefer being at home with family and friends?

At a hospital, medical aid in terms of surgery, radiation therapy, and life-monitoring machines is given. The staff is trained to handle emergency conditions, profuse bleeding, and physical care with the use of medicines, intravenous infusions, and machines to monitor bodily functions.

Is this what the terminal cancer patient needs? Perhaps. The cancer patient may require professional nursing after surgery, radiation, or during an episode of profuse bleeding or pain. However, the terminal phase of cancer is not usually medically dramatic.

What is dying from cancer like? Although it varies from person to person, the final phase for most patients is relatively quiet. Nothing more can be done or needs to be done. Medically, there is little the nurses can do except give pain shots, change an IV bottle, and take care of bodily functions for those patients who need assistance. What is needed most urgently is to keep the patient confortable and nondepressed, and usually a family member can perform this function much better than a nurse can. We tend to forget about the psychological care that is desperately needed by a person facing death. The most pressing need, according to a survey of terminal patients, is not to be abandoned by loved ones.

When we take a patient to the hospital, we expect the hospital staff to do something to allieviate the condition, to make the patient comfortable, to keep him happy. When the time of death comes, we think members of the medical profession can magically prolong life and ward off death. Or if death cannot be avoided, we expect hospital staff to handle the final moment professionally and lovingly because we who are unfamiliar with death and too close to the patient feel we will not know what to do.

Let us take a realistic look at the medical profession beginning with nurses, since they have the most contact with patients. Nurses do the best they can, and on the average they provide good medical care. They are primarily trained in hospital and medical procedures. Beyond that, they are also trained in providing emotional care. The sad truth is they do not have time to do much actual emotional counseling with patients. Most nurses care, but they just do not have time to tend to the patient's emotional needs.

Typically, nurses follow a daily plan. There is a time for medications, time for baths, time to check IVs, time to change bandages, and time to take temperature, blood pressure, and pulse. A nurse is continually busy following the schedule for her job. Nurses run in and out of the rooms in their assigned ward perhaps once every half hour or even more often stopping for a minute to perform some task. They show their caring by asking the patient how he or she is feeling.

Nurses are not callous, unfeeling creatures. Hospital costs have cut nursing staff to the bone. Nurses are overworked in hospitals that are short staffed. They work hard to accomplish their medical tasks in eight hours, to say nothing about emotional tasks. Their emotional nursing primarily consists of being nice while doing the medical tasks, but they cannot be counselors or clergymen too. Whether a nurse will be by the patient's side when death occurs is largely a matter of chance. If death happens to occur during one of the two minutes an hour when a nurse is in the room, the patient will not die alone. If the death is traumatic, numerous hospital staff will be around the bed. If the death is quiet, as most cancer deaths are, probably no one will notice when the death actually occurs.

All of us want to have a little fun at our jobs, laughing and passing our eight hours quickly. Most of us prefer jobs where we can leave the work behind us and go home without any carryovers from work.

Nurses are no different. They want to laugh at work. They also want to hurry with the paperwork so they do not have to work overtime finishing up. They have families at home and their own life away from the hospital.

A terminally ill patient is rather unpleasant for most nurses. No matter how expert the medical care, the terminal patient will die. This is very discouraging. The patient is often angry and depressed, anything but rewarding to work with. The patient's family is hurt or uncomfortable. Sometimes family members expect too much of the nurse. They want the nurse to give shots more often than the nurse is permitted to. They want the nurse to make the patient recover or to give the patient love.

Most nurses try to maintain a positive attitude toward all patients. They are at least kind. Every once in awhile a nurse will develop a special attachment to a particular patient. To love a patient who dies is painful. The nurse goes home taking her sorrow with her. Her family may feel the negative consequences of her grieving. The emotional drain is difficult on her, her family, and her effectiveness as a nurse. Soon she learns to care professionally but with distance. She protects herself from hurt.

A study shows that bells ringing in the nurses station are not all answered equally fast. Bells from terminal patients are answered slowest. Since nothing can be done medically to make a patient improve and caring will only hurt, nurses tend to avoid terminal patients. A terminal patient's depression or anger is unpleasant to deal with. Pain and discomfort the nurse cannot irradicate are hard to watch, so she doesn't.

Nurses should not be blamed for their avoidance of terminally ill patients. It makes sense when viewed from a nurse's perspective. The patient, terminal or otherwise, receives adequate medical care. Beyond that, to provide emotional care is the responsibility of the family and the people who knew and loved the patient for years previously. The nurse knows the patient for only a few days, and only eight hours of those days, and even this time is divided between many patients.

Aside from nurses, medical doctors are the main source of emotional support for a hospital patient. Doctors are hailed as all powerful healers, authority figures, decision makers, and father confessors. Patients become dependent on them for both physical and emotional needs. A period of disillusionment follows when the doctor cannot live up to these unrealistic expectations. Expecting too much in the first place explains much of the anger some people have when their doctors turn out to be mere humans who cannot perform miracles and even have their own needs.

What can reasonably be expected from a doctor? Primarily medical skills, since this is what they are trained to do. If you are looking for emotional support or problem resolution guidance, a medical doctor may not be what you need: a psychologist or mental health counselor is more skilled in these areas. Some medical doctors treat diseases first, people second. Perhaps this is the way it should be, since an M.D.'s training is in medicine and not in emotional support. You initially choose a doctor on the basis of his or her skill in a disease or treatment area. Is it fair to change the rules of the game midstream and start to expect something else? If your doctor gives you emotional support, you are getting something extra above and beyond what you have a right to expect.

Some doctors are very good with patients. They have a warm and friendly bedside manner, listening to the patient's fears and treating the emotional correlates of the disease. Most doctors have some of this quality in them, but some obviously have more than others. It is easier to be warm and friendly when the doctor knows he or she can help the patient. Some pediatricians tickle and play with a cooing baby whose ear infection is easily cured. It is much harder to be relaxed and jovial with the child whose leukemia will not go into remission and who instead becomes weaker with each visit. The doctor has his or her own sadness to handle as well as the illness.

Some of the emotional distance also called "professionalism" is due to training. Doctors were drilled in the fields of anatomy, physiology, pathology, and so forth. In contrast, a Ph.D. psychologist has spent his or her university years studying the emotional side of people and how relationships work to fulfill psychological needs.

Besides training, the way a doctor relates to patients depends to some extent on his own psychological style or personality. The authoritarian doctor will make the decisions for the patient. This kind of doctor may withhold upsetting information. Less authoritarian doctors will tell you the pros and cons of a situation and let you decide which way to go. The authoritarian doctor feels he has many years of medical school and residency behind his decision. The democratic kind of doctor feels you have a right to participate in the decisions made about your body. Most doctors will truthfully answer a question when it is put to them straight but are hesitant about supplying more information than requested.

The patient often has to know which questions to ask.

Doctors and nurses are overworked, especially if they are good. Primarily this is due not to a desire to make lots of money. Rather, it is because good doctors get many referrals from other doctors, former patients, and just general knowledge about "Who is good." It is hard for a doctor to turn a patient away when he believes in himself and his ability to help a patient who might otherwise suffer.

It can be frustrating to attempt communication with some doctor who is gruff, busy, and unskilled in ministering emotional concerns. It would be nice to have a doctor with the nurturant manner of a television doctor and the skills of a great healer who never lost a patient. Unfortunately, it is not likely to happen very often. Most people are left with the tasks of finding doctors who are highly skilled in their medical specialty and coping with their interpersonal style however unrewarding it may be.

As young children our first experience with pain was that someone we loved could make the hurt go away. If a finger was injured, tears brought a parent who kissed the finger and made the pain disappear. When we were punished for misbehavior and promised to be good, the pain was also alleviated.

When pain strikes a cancer patient, there is often regression to these earlier modes of interaction. The patient wants someone to make him feel better and to take away the cancer. Sometimes the patient feels guilty for having contracted cancer and wants to be relieved of the blame. When he is reaching out for compassion, sometimes there is no one to help.

In a hospital, nurses want to help and often do, but they have a whole ward of people who are sick and in pain. Doctors are with the patient for only a few minutes a day. A doctor can prescribe pain medication, conduct surgery, order radiation, things that actually involve doing a lot to control pain. Sometimes they cannot do everything the way an all-powerful parent could for a young child.

Frequently, the doctor's response to a patient's pain seems rather matter-of-fact. This may be because the doctor has seen other cases that are similar, so he or she does not need to ponder which course of action to take. Also the doctor may have other terminal or sad cases weighing heavy on his mind. If you think the doctor looks preoccupied, you might be right.

To most doctors, death is failure. They are trained and dedicated to life. In reality an unhappy death is sad; a peaceful accepting death is success. Nobody avoids death forever.

Some doctors preserve life at all costs and under all circumstances. No matter how diminished in capacity a patient is, some doctors think any kind of life is worthwhile. In terminal phases of life, that choice ought to be the patient's. Life when one cannot talk, remember, move, or take care of bodily functions is just not worth living for some people.

If you want some choice about what kind of suffering you have to go through in the name of treatment and want to be able to say "Enough!" and let nature take its course, then your most important task is to find a doctor who agrees with you. You need a doctor who will work with you and keep you comfortable if all else fails.

Do not expect the doctor to feel good about having a patient who is going to die. But do keep searching until you find a competent specialist who will loyally hang in there with the patient to the end, combining his expertise with the patient's preferences about what kind of life is worth living.

All of these things are possible at home. Physical care of a cancer patient is manageable without nursing training. All medications including narcotics for pain can be administered at home with a little training. Many more techniques besides shots can be learned to alleviate pain.

The emotional aspects of terminal cancer must be dealt with whether or not the patient is in the hospital. There is no pill that can make the situation go away. However, at home the environment is much more conducive to working through the intense emotions both the patient and the family are feeling.

Remember that hospitals and hospices are money-making businesses. They must remain solvent to stay in operation, whether they are run by religious orders or corporations. Your loved one is just one of many who pass through their doors.

Dying at home may not be for everyone, but a person should always investigate all alternatives before making a choice. Probably the most important consideration should be where the cancer patient wants to spend his or her last days; what does he want to look at, what does he want to remember?

What, then, can you expect from hospitals and nurses? You can expect good medical care. Hospitals handle emergencies, operations, and laboratory tests. When there is nothing more the hospital can do, it is time to go home. What you have a right to expect the hospital and the medical staff to provide is itemized on your bill. You will not find love on the list.

CONTENTS

DYING AT HOME
WITH CANCER

Chapter 1

CHOOSING TO DIE AT HOME

WHERE should the terminally ill patient spend his last days to get the physical and emotional care he or she needs? In most cases, there comes a point when the hospital can do nothing more medically. In the final phase of cancer, usually all that is done physically is to give pain injections. Time must be passed until death.

During this final stage of the illness, the patient has many emotional needs, perhaps more than at any previous stage of life. These emotional needs involve coming to grips with dying and realizing that the family can manage afterwards. The patient needs to look around his home, see the children, work at hobbies, and feel that his existence was not in vain. One must see the fruits of life's labor.

Feeling secure is a primary need. The patient must know someone will be there to help him if he has pain or feels lonely. There are many things that can be done to alleviate pain in addition to giving a shot. However, someone must be willing to spend time with the patient.

At home you have control of all aspects of a patient's care and can make decisions in the patient's best interest. Not only do you control when pain medication is given, you can decide whether life-prolonging measures such as respirators are going to be used. Visitors can be scheduled at the patient's convenience rather than the hospital's. Uncomfortable hospital procedures can be halted.

Modern culture sells fear of death. Youth and beauty are emulated. Movies and magaizines show us that the world is populated only by people who are young, healthy, and beautiful. Natural death is no longer thought of as a family affair. Grandmother is not expected to live with her daughter's family. She is expected to go away to a retirement community. When it is time to die, she is expected to do it quickly and neatly in a hospital or politely in her sleep.

A person with a terminal illness poses a threat to this type of culture. Death is supposed to be quick, neat, and conducted out of sight. Lingering upsets people by rocking the myths of youth, health, and beauty. To solve this dilemma, terminal patients are shut up in antiseptic hospital rooms away from the sight of family and friends. Usually no one under age sixteen is permitted in terminal wards. This leaves out the grandchildren and younger children to whom the patient wants to say good-bye.

Hospital rooms are uncomfortable places for people to visit. Chairs are either absent or lack upholstering. With all of the apparatus surrounding the high hospital bed, visitors huddle in the corners looking up at a distance to the patient. There is nothing to look at, nowhere to move to. The physical setup coupled with nurses walking in and out makes any meaningful communication impossible.

Dying patients need more than flowers or an occasional visitor. They need to come to grips with dying. They may need to talk about death and what their life has meant.

Terminally ill patients initially fear dying. Even more, the patients fear dying alone, isolated from people who care. Someone is quoted who said we come into the world alone and have to go out of the world alone. This need not be true. A person who is loved does not have to die alone if his family cares enough to remain at his side.

The family of the terminal patient has emotional issues to be resolved. Some must tell the patient that the past slights are forgiven. Others need to ask for forgiveness while there is still time. Most want to tell the patient how important he or she is. The patient needs to be reassured that should living become too difficult, it is all right to go. This kind of communication is practically impossible in a hospital room where family members are herded in a corner 10 feet from the patient and next to the roommate's visitors.

Contrast the situation at home. The patient is resting in the bedroom or living room he spent years enjoying. Surrounding the patient are treasured mementos of a full life. On the wall there are knick-knacks from vacations and pictures of the kids. The familiar scene out the window viewed so many times is comforting. Not even a hospice can offer this.

Visitors can come and go as the patient requests. The patient can listen to his favorite music. Hearing is the last sense to go it is said, but what is there to hear in the hospital but the preselected pop radio stations or the clatter of dinner trays going down the hall?

At home, when death comes, the patient will not be alone or with strangers. A family member will be at his bedside holding his hand. When lonely or in pain he knows someone will come running. If he wants to die with dignity when the time comes, no hospital orderly is going to resuscitate him with a machine.

Benefits of Home Care

Even with the added work, the benefits of home care outweigh the convenience of hospital care for both the patient and the family. The advantages occur in many areas: cost, availability of pain medication, dignity, comfort, security, and a chance for everyone involved to work through their emotions.

Many terminal cancer patients worry since their hospice or hospital stay eats up a lifetime of savings intended to help the family. Costs can be drastically cut by dying at home. Equipment rental can be kept to a minimum. You can get by adequately without a hospital bed, commode, and wheelchair or borrow them gratis from an agency like the American Cancer Society.

All medications can be administered at home by the family even if you have no nursing background. All you need is an agreeable doctor who will work out arrangements to get narcotics. Needles are disposable these days so sterilization is not needed; usually, the whole syringe is thrown away after each injection. Since the syringes come assembled, all you have to do is put the medicine in the arm. Morphine is a little bit more complicated because the syringe must be inserted into the metal tubex frame, but still the needle is disposable.

Toilet functions are sometimes a concern. As long as the patient is mobile, he or she will manage going to the bathroom. Later you can use a bedpan. Since cancer patients eat and drink progressively less and less, there is not as much waste as with a healthy person. Incontinence may be a problem in some atypical cases. You can try to catheterize the patient or to condition him to eliminate at a certain time, but possibly you may just change sheets often. For the other kind of problem, constipation, enemas can be administered while the patient is in bed. So even with the various elimination problems, bedridden patients do not have to be carried around; everything can be handled while they remain in bed.

With bathing, the situation is the same. Continue tub baths as long as the patient can get around. Rather than lifting an incapacitated patient in and out of the tub, switch to sponge baths in bed.

A lot is said these days about dying with dignity. This means being treated like a respected and loved person, not just like another case. There is no way to provide this kind of loving care except at home, or perhaps at a special cancer hospice, providing the family stays there also. You have no way of insuring that a life ready to end is not being artificially prolonged except at home where you control what is done. When to give a shot is your choice at home. You do not have to search for a nurse, wait for her to answer the light, and then be told the patient must still wait a while longer. At home the patient remains in his own clothes, in his own environment, talking to people he knows who treat him with respect. This is real dignity, not dying in a hospital gown open down the back.

Another benefit to keeping a loved one at home is that you can take better care of yourself. You can change clothes, sleep in your bed, wash your hair and eat the healthy food you are accustomed to. Food from hospital vending machines will not keep you going long. At home you have the props that make all of you comfortable: pictures of the kids, the family pet, the restful scene from the windows.

The arguments against home care mainly revolve around the fact that it is tiring and demanding. Having a loved one die of cancer is demanding whether he or she dies at home or in a hospital. There is no easy way out. At least at home, you can do it your way.

A family goes through a lot when one of its members dies. Cancer is especially feared. The family agonizes about what the end will be like for their loved one. Keeping a terminally ill patient at home when the hospital can do nothing more provides the family with the opportunity to work through the grieving process. It gives the family a chance to help the patient while he needs help. No one else can do what the family can. Nurses and doctors provide medical treatment. Family members provide emotional treatment. Providing care helps the family accept the death, work through the grief, and eliminate guilt feelings that naturally occur during living.

My father died of terminal cancer that began as lung cancer. Later he developed small intestine cancer that metastasized to his liver. He spent over six months in bed before he died.

Dad went to the hospital a few times during those months for emergencies. The hospital took care of the acute problem, and he went home again with the chronic and incurable problem. The last time he went to the hospital he was very frightened. He knew he was getting weaker, and he feared he would not leave the hospital. When he voiced this fear, we worked quickly to take him home.

My family learned how and when to give shots. We also learned how to operate the nasal-gastric pump that helped keep him comfortable by removing distending fluids. We took him home and cared for him until he died a peaceful and, under the circumstances, happy man. Dad was comfortable about dying and so were the rest of us. When it was time, we let him go with love. He actually kissed us moments before he died.

Losing someone to a terminal disease is not easy. But a powerful experience such as this has the potential to be either very uplifting or very dangerous to you emotionally. After my experience with my father, I saw terminally ill patients and their families in my private practice as a psychologist. Families who cared for loved ones at home had far less grief to work through than families whose loved one died alone one night at the hospital.

In our personal case, my family was very sorry when Dad died, but we did not feel that crippling anguish about his parting that others exhibited at the funeral. We knew what he had gone through. We also knew we had diminished his discomfort, serving him during his greatest need.

We had the opportunity to watch Dad accept his own dying. At the end he was not angry or depressed as he had been earlier. We also shared the peace of acceptance that came as a result of talking with him about his dying and helping make it a successful part of living.

Sometimes in my practice, I see family members who are visibly, physically suffering anguish years and years after a loved one dies. In most of these cases, the loss was sudden. Sometimes there was a period of suffering in a hospital. Some of these survivors spend years in therapy talking to an empty chair saying all the things they should have said to the dying person.

What This Book Can Offer

This book tells how to care for a terminally ill patient at home when family members have no medical training. Most of my work is with cancer patients, so I concentrate on the particular experiences and procedures that go along with cancer. The same procedures would work with other kinds of terminal illnesses or plain old age with some variations.

The physical procedures done in the hospital can usually be followed at home with little or no training. Whatever training is needed can be picked up by watching nurses at the hospital or getting training in the doctor's office. The emotional care cannot be provided in the hospital by nurses. Family members can provide emotional care anyplace, although it is easiest to do in your home where you and the patient are comfortable. What to say about death and why to say it are explained. There are several stages leading to the final stage of acceptance of death. This book illustrates how to handle each stage, giving examples of what to say or not to say. Since the final stage of acceptance is a comfortable stage to be in for the family and the patient, I suggest ways to reach this stage and how to work out of the less comfortable stages of depression and anger.

Talking about dying is difficult at first. Thinking about what to say is the most difficult part. After the topic is first broached, conversing about death becomes easier. Hints to help the patient get his feelings out are provided, along with suggestions for family members who seem to be having a difficult time dealing with the pending death. Also, techniques for communicating your feelings on the topic of death and dying are given.

Symptoms for gauging how close to death the patient is are presented along with an idea of what the death may be like. While no one can tell you exactly how your loved one will die, I try to give you an idea of what you are getting into when you take someone home to die.

Since pain control is of paramount importance to cancer patients, I go into various methods of pain control to provide more options in and greater understanding of the procedures available for alleviating discomfort. The most often used pain medications available for cancer patients are described; for example, how the dosages are escalated, what happens when drugs are combined, and whether you have to worry about drug dependence and addiction. From this discussion you will better understand the drug plan the physician works out for the patient and you will be able to discuss changes if the medication is not sufficient.

Techniques for the administration of pain medication are described in detail; for example, how to give shots and where on the body to give them are explained for the person who has never given a shot before.

Sometimes cancer patients need some kind of life-supporting device. Suggestions are given on how to operate the common ones, what equipment you may have to rent, and what you can do without. Moral and personal issues surrounding the dilemma of whether to disconnect these devices at a certain point or not are discussed.

Also presented are legal measures the patient can take while healthy to specify the kind of care he or she wants while still living. I provide an example of such a document already legal in many states. You can have the patient fill out the form indicating the limits of the care to be provided or giving the decision-making power to a trusted family member or friend.

This book is dedicated to the proposition that the cancer patient with a terminal diagnosis still has various options available to make the final phase of living comfortable, physically and emotionally. Dying at home may not be for everyone, but it may be the best choice for most people. I have been through it with my father and many times assisting other families. It can be one of the most worthwhile experiences in your life. The physical care is easy to learn. The emotional care of the patient and of yourself is something you will have to manage whether the patient dies at home or in a hospital. So let us roll up our sleeves and make the best of the situation!

Chapter 2

PROVIDING NURSING CARE

THERE is nothing mysterious or magical about nursing someone, particularly a cancer patient. You can learn all the
necessary skills by watching the hospital staff and asking a few
questions. This chapter provides suggestions for providing general
care. For unusual procedures, training from a nurse will be necessary.

If your relative is at the hospital, have everyone from the
family who is going to provide nursing care remain in the hospital
room all day for a day or two. Ask the nurses to show you how to
do everything they do. The first day they will show you; the
second day ask them to watch you perform the task.

I found the nurses to be extremely helpful in this teaching
task. Nurses generally agree terminal cancer patients are better
off at home with their families than in a hospital. They gladly
demonstrate procedures and make lists of things to remember.

*During the terminal stages of his illness, my father was afraid
of being alone, so we decided to bring home to the hospital until
we could take him home for good. Home is people and treasured
possessions. We paired off in shifts around the clock keeping conversation going in between. Photo albums of happy times helped
us remember. Dad liked to listen and would laugh at the proper
moments, but he could not talk much himself.*

*We had to take care of ourselves, too. From home we brought
in some nutritious food to sustain us over the long hours. The
nurses gave mother a rollaway bed so she could stretch out at
night. This was typical of their hospitality and willingness to have*

us stay around the clock with Dad.

Dad was delighted to have us remain with him. Saying that someone who is going to die needs his rest is usually an excuse to get away. When Dad wanted to sleep, he said so, and we all settled down for a snooze. When he wanted to talk, we talked, even if it was in the middle of the night. We shut the door to Dad's private room and tried to be as unobtrusive as possible so as not to bother other patients. We succeeded in bringing home to the hospital and had a good time while doing it.

Some of the areas you need expertise in include how to prepare foods that are on the patient's diet, how to give shots and operate the machines that make the patient feel comfortable, how to select the appropriate enema and give it to a bedridden patient, how to deal with catheters and incontinence, and how to care for a bedridden person's body.

Food

The decisions about food revolve around the doctor's decision to rule out certain kinds of food, such as solids when the intestines are blocked. After the doctor has determined what is out, the patient can impose his likes or dislikes and choose what he feels like eating from the list of possible foods. You can help by preparing attractive and varied food from the list of eligibles. Also, you can be creative and think of unusual or different ways of preparing the food, especially important when the choices are limited and the same food has to be offered very often. In general, when you ask the patient what he wishes for lunch, give him a choice between two foods on the list. Say, "Would you like broth or jello?" rather than "What would you like for lunch?" What the patient wants and what the patient can have are usually two different things.

Cancer patients go through taste changes as the cancer progresses. One common change is a dislike of meat. The smell and taste of even old favorite entrees make the patient nauseated.

Mother could not bake the Thanksgiving turkey at home for the first time in over thirty years because Dad could not tolerate the aroma. As the cancer progressed, it became increasingly difficult to find food Dad would eat. His appetite diminished dramatically. Then his intestines became partially blocked, so he had to go on a liquid diet. A canned liquid protein supplement became his primary staple.

When most people imagine a liquid diet, they think of coffee, tea, broth, and jello, which are pretty boring. We found many other foods to add to this list.

Herbal teas for example, are available in many flavors. For variety they can be served iced or hot, with or without sweetner. Herbal teas are generally not caffeinated unless you get a kind whose name implies stimulation, such as "Morning Thunder." Camomile tea is very soothing and relaxing. It can be given at night to help a restless patient drift into sleep. Comfrey tea is supposed to clear the mucus out of the intestine by acting like a mild laxative. Peppermint tea and rosehips tea provide refreshing flavors and some vitamins. Your local health store has many kinds, either loose or in tea bags, with a description of what the tea contains. For the patient who needs to intake a certain amount of fluids, clear tea is virtually the same as water.

An older couple I worked with began having afternoon tea when the wife was bedridden with cancer. Between three and four every afternoon, she combed her hair and donned a frilly bed jacket. Her husband, who was retired and attended her all day, changed shirts and helped her into a wheelchair. Then he brought in their best sterling silver tea service on a tray with two bone china cups and a single flower in a bud vase. For the next half hour, they shared formal tea and discussed matters unrelated to sickness. After tea, she returned to bed. This tea ritual became a treasured high point in their day. Although they no longer went out, they escaped from the illness into a civilized activity each day. She died at home very contentedly with the help of her elderly husband who, by the way, still takes tea every afternoon in remembrance of his wife.

If the patient likes coffee, for variety try expresso or decaffeinated coffee, coffee with wheat added, chicory coffee, or the new international flavors on the market. If you use a fancy tea service with tea, try using mugs with coffee. The variety of a restricted diet is limited, so there must be variety in the way food is served.

Another food that added variety to the liquid diet is fruit juice. There are many fruit juices: orange, apple, pear, peach, papaya, grapefruit, grape, to name only a few. You will have to strain the juice through cheesecloth to remove all the pulp. Canned baby apple and orange juice is already strained so it can pass through a baby bottle nipple.

Again, how juices are served makes a difference. Glasses and cups of various shapes can be iced in the freezer and placed on a doily, which rests on a plate. Fancy or plastic twisted straws, swiggle sticks, or paper parasols can be inserted to make it look more decorative and cheerful.

You may freeze juices to make refreshing popsicles. When frozen juice is blended you create an ice slush similar to sherbet. Sometimes the patient is able to eat commercial sherbet, which adds a desertlike quality to meals.

Clear broth need not be as boring as it sounds. Any number of canned broths are commercially available. You can make broths in a crock pot or pressure cooker as well as on the stove. Check with your doctor for sure, but most patients can eat soup made from any vegetable, seasoning, meat or fish, as long as the particles of food are strained out with a sieve or cheesecloth. Strain it for the patient and eat the food part yourself. You must not forget to take care of yourself while caring for another.

On a liquid diet, milk is not permitted because it becomes a solid in the stomach. Therefore, do not make cream soup or vichyssoise. Do not serve ice cream or frozen yogurt for the same reason.

Besides sherbet and frozen juice, jello is another desert permitted on a liquid diet. Jello molds made with fruit juice are attractive and refreshing. Jello can be whipped before it is completely set to give it a pleasant texture and the appearance of added whipped cream.

Other foods for diversion and to put a pleasant taste in the mouth are hard candies and mints. Be careful the patient does not recline with a hard candy in his or her mouth for fear of getting it stuck in the airway. Cancer patients really enjoy a spray of breath freshener or mouth wash for breath refreshment.

In conclusion, as far as food goes, work around the doctor's orders. Serve food attractively. Try variations of hot and cold. When friends call and offer to help, tell them the dietary restrictions and see if they can come up with creative alternatives you did not think of. Also keep in mind that cancer naturally distorts the sensation of taste, so pretty soon nothing except certain cold drinks tastes good. At that point try various flavors of soda pop, fruit juices, and herbal teas.

Since the cancer patient is the one who is most intimately experiencing the ordeal, he deserves to make some of the choices and maintain control over his body. Force feeding is cruel. Intravenous feedings, known as IVs, provide liquid and some nourishment, but they also prolong life. When providing care, do your best regarding food and liquids and leave the rest up to the patient. Adult patients understand the consequences. If the patient can accept these consequences, we should also.

Pumps and IVs

An IV, intravenous fluid, is an inverted bottle of fluid hung above the patient on a stand connected to the patient by a needle inserted into a vein. Arm veins are the first choice. When they are overused, other veins are found on the body. An IV provides fluids for the body, as well as nourishment and vitamins. An IV can remain in one location for about three days before the vein becomes damaged.

Hospital staff routinely insert IVs because they provide quick access for putting medication into the blood stream. In a cancer patient, like any other kind of patient, IVs serve to prolong life. Once an IV is taken out of a patient who is getting no fluids by mouth, the body cannot survive very long, since toxins build up in already weak organs.

Besides the IV, an N-G, which is a nasal-gastric pump, is frequently used. A rubber tube is inserted into the nose and run down into the stomach. The tube is connected to a pump, which provides suction to pull up fluids that accumulate in the stomach. These fluids are both natural stomach juices and any liquids received orally. The fluids collect in a glass tube that has to be emptied daily. The purpose of an N-G is to keep the stomach clear of fluids because with the obstruction below the stomach, there is nowhere for the fluids to go. Instead they collect in the stomach, distend or push out the stomach, and create pain.

For comfort's sake, Dad's N-G was kept operating until the end. It did not prolong life; it just kept him comfortable. When Dad got thirsty, he took liquids by mouth. The doctor said we could unplug the N-G to give the fluids a chance to be absorbed while in the stomach, but since Dad expressly requested not to prolong this phase of his life, we kept the N-G operating all the time. So he took in liquids to keep his mouth wet and the pump immediately took them out.

Operating the N-G was easy to learn. The tube never came out of the nose. We kept the suction going at the setting prescribed by the doctor. Twice a day the jar had to be emptied and the volume of the contents recorded on the output chart.

At first I must admit being rather taken aback by the color of the discharge. Usually, it was dark amber colored with small dark flecks. Of course, when Dad drank strained orange juice (strained to keep out any pulp that might clog the tubes), orange was what came out of the tube.

The tube has to be kept clear. With a large syringe, warm water is inserted into the tube running to the stomach to backwash the tubes. The water immediately runs out, taking any clots or particles that might plug the tube. If the tube resisted unplugging, dissolving a teaspoon of baking soda in a couple of cups of lukewarm water and using a scant fourth cup (30 cc) of this solution to backwash usually unplugs the tube.

If the tube is not extracting as it should, two problems need to be investigated. Are the tubes unplugged? Is the lid on the jar tightly to maintain proper suction? Also check that the machine is set on the proper degree of suction. Frequently, intermittent suction is preferred over continuous suction, which is sometimes too hard on the stomach.

Most companies that rent the N-G have repair representatives available twenty-four hours a day by beeper. If the unit malfunctions, they promise a replacement within an hour. Check that the company you rent from makes a similar agreement.

Enemas

Bedridden patients or patients with cancer of the abdomen may require an occasional enema to avoid becoming plugged up.

Contemplating the giving of an enema is worse than actually doing it. The situation is analogous to changing your own baby's messy diaper, which is not so bad as opposed to someone else's baby whose mess smells somehow foreign.

Enemas can be given to the patient in bed. Place a towel or plastic sheet under the patient's bottom to protect the bed. Put the patient lying on his or her back with a bed pan under the buttocks. The bed can be flat or tilted up to an almost sitting position. Some people prefer giving an enema to a patient on a bed pan while reclining in a bathtub or sitting on a commode.

Another bed position is to place the patient half on his stomach, half on his side, with one leg bent and pulled up toward the waist. A pillow put under the abdomen and another under the head and arms makes the patient more comfortable. With this position, the enema will be conducted while the bag is held five to fifteen inches above the rectum. The patient will roll over onto his back to sit on the bed pan before dispelling the contents.

Various kinds of enema solutions are available. The easiest and most expensive are the already prepared solutions available in drug stores. Most come in a disposable applicator.

You can make your own enema solutions. The solution should be lukewarm, not over 105 degrees Fahrenheit to avoid burning the delicate rectal membrane. You can use plain tap water or a saline enema made by dissolving 1 teaspoon of salt into 1 pint of tap water. Salt is used to maintain the delicate electrolytic balance of the body, which can be upset by frequent enemas. Dissolving one ounce of pure soap solution in one quart of water is another possibility, although this kind of enema should be used cautiously, since soap is harsh on the rectum and promotes vigorous muscle contractions. The doctor may order a special enema such as a mineral oil preparation, which makes expelling the feces a little easier. The same procedure is followed except that the oil is usually not heated but rather is used at room temperature.

Regardless of the kind of solution used, the procedure to follow is the same. Prepare the enema and lubricate the tip with vaseline, cold cream, or lotion. Put the patient into position and have the bed pan ready. Toilet paper and warm wet washclothes should be within reach. Lubricate the anus with vaseline and .

gently insert the applicator. Use an enema applicator, not one used for another purpose such as douching. Do not push the applicator too deep or too roughly. However, the applicator has to be inserted deep enough that it will stay in place.

The solution must be given slowly so as not to hurt the colon or give the patient discomfort. Hold the enema bag up above the rectum, five to fifteen inches. No higher or the fluid will enter too quickly given the pull of gravity. Open the catch that closes the tube and squeeze the enema bag.

How much solution to put in depends. If the patient reports discomfort, stop. If the doctor says a certain amount must be given during one enema, start and stop the flow until the entire amount is taken in. Cramps will usually cease if you stop the flow momentarily.

Sometimes the doctor orders the inserted fluids be retained for up to thirty minutes. This is to soften the feces and to relieve gas. Insert the entire amount all at once or by the start and stop method. Begin timing when the fluid is all in the body. Dispel at the end of the elapsed time.

The most usual procedure is that the contents of the enema are supposed to be dispelled as soon as the patient wants. In the unlikely event that the contents are not dispelled within thirty minutes, call your doctor, since this may be a sign of an internal disorder.

Sometimes feces are so impacted that they cannot be dispelled by a single enema. The resulting blockage causes the patient pain when the intestines go into spasm trying to dispel the hard mass. When this happens, give the patient a muscle relaxant before trying repeated enemas. Also, you may try different kinds of solutions such as mineral oil or warm soapy water to soften the blockage from the bottom. From the top, have the patient take a laxative. You can also try inserting a glycerin suppository into the rectum. It will stimulate vigorous muscle contractions, which may move the mass.

If you try everything and the fecal mass will not move or if the patient is in much pain, call your doctor. It may be time for the patient to go to the hospital for a day or two in order to get cleaned out.

Some foods are constipating and should be avoided if constipation is a problem. They include bananas, yogurt, and bland foods. Fresh fruits and vegetables, anything hard to chew, are better. The real culprits are lack of exercise and bland foods. You may not be able to do anything about these factors given the disease. You can try 100% bran cereal with a prune juice chaser late in the evening just before retiring. They usually work better at night to push through all the food eaten during the day than if given in the morning. You can also ask your doctor for diet changes if constipation continues to be a problem. The patient may end up on a liquid diet.

Catheters and Incontinence

Some cancer patients are unable to hold their urine or their bowel movements. Sometimes this is due to being overmedicated. Usually, if this is going to happen, it happens toward the end, but not all patients have this problem. The inability to control these functions is called incontinence.

The problems with incontinence are twofold: there is a problem with the patient and a problem for the caretakers. The patient must be kept clean and dry or else bed sores, which are painful and hard to cure, can develop. This means if the patient is continually leaking, he must be frequently washed. Bedding must be changed often.

The problem for the caretakers is having to deal constantly with feces. The smell and the laundry can wear a caretaker down.

To minimize laundry you can try putting a rubber sheet crossways on the bed under the patient. Then you need something to catch the excrement. Paper towels or flat open disposable diapers work well. As often as you clean up a leak, you will have to wash and dry the patient.

You can try conditioning the patient to expel his urine and feces at a certain time. For a day or two, mark down the times of day when the accidents occur. Do they always occur within five minutes of giving a drink? If so, put the patient on the commode before giving him a drink. When you hear the patient wet, say "Good, Sam. You are passing urine." The patient needs to pair his sensation of voiding with whatever senses or feelings he has at that moment so he can recognize when he needs to go to the bathroom.

Sometimes you condition yourself by just recognizing those times when the patient is likely to have to eliminate. Then you make sure you have him on the commode in time.

With bowel incontinence you can try using a glycerin suppository to bring down the feces when you have the patient on the commode. This will not work with diarrhea, which tends to come often.

For urinary incontinence, you could ask the doctor about a catheter. A catheter is a drainage tube passed into the bladder through the urethra. It allows for continuous drainage of urine through the tube into a rubber bag. It is usually used to obtain an uncontaminated urine specimen for a test or for surgery patients who are unable to pass urine at all or cannot hold it back.

The way a catheter is inserted is that a doctor or nurse puts the tubing into a well-cleaned urethra and pushes it up into the bladder. Once the tube is in place, a little balloon on the tip of the tube inside the bladder is inflated with water. The balloon serves to keep the tube from working its way out of the bladder. If the tubing is jerked when the balloon is inflated, damage can be done to the bladder.

The Foley catheter used generally on women is held in place by the inflated balloon. But if the tube should be inadvertently pulled, there can be injury to the patient by putting pressure on the bladder. To avoid this, some people tape the tube to the patient's leg using the surgical tape, which does not hurt when pulled off, or putting a pin around the tube and attaching it to the bedding or the pajamas can be tried.

Some catheters have no balloon. They are used only for a short time, either to obtain a urine specimen or if the patient cannot void. The external catheter is a thin plastic sheath that fits over a man's penis. It is held in place with tape or a special fastener.

If an external catheter is used, ask for a demonstration of how the external catheter is fastened to the penis. Then you can check your patient frequently to make sure that it is not on too tight. You can tell if it is too tight because the penis will become swollen or look dark red to black if the blood circulation is cut off. If this happens, the external catheter has to be loosened.

Insertion and maintenance of a catheter are sterile procedures, since bacteria readily grow in the warm environment of the bladder. Sterile gloves are worn, and all the equipment must be sterile. Irrigation of the catheter, which involves inserting fluid up the catheter into the bladder to wash it out, must also be conducted under clean conditions.

Although it is unusual, sometimes a confused patient will try to pull out the tube. You can keep the patient from reaching the tube by tucking a sheet tightly around the hips. Or tuck the sheet in tightly under the armpits with the hands out, again so the patient cannot reach the tube. As a last resort you can try Posey mitts or Posey limb holders, which are comfortable restraints that tie the patient's hands to the side of the bed. Most cancer patients do not need restraints because they are coherent enough to understand what they are doing.

You should check that the catheter is draining continuously. The tube should not be clamped or kinked, nor should the patient have pain or swelling in the lower abdomen from a bladder filled with urine. Never let the urine drain back into the bladder from the collection bag. The urine should never touch the end of the tube because bacteria can infiltrate up the tube into the bladder, causing infection. Having your patient drink a lot of fluids helps keep the bladder cleaned out. Cranberry juice is especially good for preventing bacteria growth in the bladder.

Backrubs

The need for backrubs and just touching cannot be overemphasized. Touch the patient constantly. Someone should always be sitting right next to the bed stroking an arm. Family and friends can take turns even when the patient is comatose. Bodily contact is more important than small talk.

Beyond the need for human contact through touching, backrubs serve the purpose of toughening the skin and stimulating circulation. They also get the patient turned over. The movement in bed is very important to keep muscles in tone. Backrubs should be given every two to four hours. A good backrub takes about two to three minutes.

You can vary the substance you apply to the skin during the backrub. Possibilities are lotion, powder, alcohol, cornstarch, or a mixture of alcohol and oil. Sometimes the heavily perfumed substances should be avoided, since some cancer patients strongly dislike any odor.

When you give a backrub, rub the skin gently without scratching, yet firmly. Use large, relaxing circular movements. Do not pound the skin the way Swedish masseuses do unless your patient requests it, and even then show discretion.

It is suggested that the legs not be rubbed because circulation is so poor in the extremeties of bedridden patients that clots form. Rubbing loosens these clots, which can then travel in the bloodstream and potentially plug a vessel elsewhere.

However, other places on the body can be rubbed. Places showing redness or other signs of wear should receive special attention before they get worse.

The skin over Dad's hip bones and tailbones looked red at the pressure points where most of the weight of the body rested. We carefully and gently rubbed these areas very often, sometimes every hour, and tried to turn Dad frequently to give the skin a rest. Where Dad's ankles rubbed against the sheets, the skin looked worn and the feet were very cold. Once we applied down-filled booties, the feet stayed warmer. The skin never completely healed, but at least it did not get worse. Dad never had broken skin bedsores, and for someone in bed for over six months, I think that's pretty good.

Any hand movement technique you develop will be fine for backrubs. One particularly restful technique is to pour lotion in your hands and use long, smooth strokes from the buttocks to the shoulders. Circular movements can be employed over any reddened areas.

Remember to watch your own posture while bending forward over the bed. Reaching out for three minutes puts a lot of pressure on your back muscles. Put your legs as close to the patient's bed as possible with one foot in front of the other. The bed should be raised high so you do not have to bend over so much. Stand near the buttocks and push your arms up toward the patient's neck.

If the bed is wide, it will be easier to rub each side of the body separately, moving from one side of the bed to the other.

Backrubs should be pleasant times for the patient and the caregiver. A backrub is so relaxing that it will help the patient go to sleep. If the patient experiences some pain but not enough to warrant a pain shot, a backrub can supply the relaxing diversion necessary to help the patient cope with the discomfort.

Useful Equipment and Supplies to Rent, Buy, or Make

There are any number of devices and equipment that you can rent. Every object you see in a hospital room can be rented: bed, tray, commode, wheelchair, oxygen, pumps. You can probably get by with much less equipment than the hospital has, so choose only those objects that will really help you to provide good care.

The motorized hospital beds as opposed to the crank type are easiest to operate but also the costliest to rent. The crank hospital bed does all the same things as the motorized version: the head and legs fold and the whole bed goes up and down, but you supply the power by turning a crank at the foot of the bed. The crank turns easily, and only a couple of turns are needed to raise the head of the bed full up. The mattresses come protected by a plastic cover, which has been sanitized.

Hospital equipment and supplies in the yellow pages lists many rental businesses. Often they deliver at no charge, provide free home evaluations, and repair or replace equipment on a twenty-four hour basis. Besides beds, you can rent or buy tables that can be raised or lowered and pushed over the bed. Also available are wheelchairs, walkers, patient lifts, bath lifts, walkers and crutches, commodes, ostomy supplies, special cushions, stair and porch elevators, car hand controls, much more than you will ever need. All that is mandatory is a pump or any machine the patient needs to control fluids for comfort or oxygen for breathing. You will probably have to buy a bedpan. Although the specific needs of each patient vary, you will probably not need to rent much equipment. The objects you will have to buy are even fewer.

You can make objects to help keep the patient more comfortable. If you have a friend or relative who wants to do something for you, let him or her make some of these objects. It is important to get concerned people involved.

My sister Bonnie made sheepskin covers for Dad's elbows, knees, and ankles. To do this, take a piece of sheepskin, natural is better than synthetic, and cut out a piece like a circle. Then cut out a piece like a piece of pie from the circle. Stitch the circle together along the edge of the cut out piece to make a cone. Try it in paper first so you will know how big a circle to cut. The cone fits over the elbow. It can be held in place by ribbons or self-adhesive materials. For the ankles and knees, a larger flat piece of sheepskin, soft side turned in, works well.

Cutting off the toes of soft socks makes fine pullovers for elbows, knees and ankles, if you do not want to bother with the sheepskin. I liked the stockinette pullovers because they could be easily laundered and were not obtrusive.

Bedding is important for health and comfort. Always use unstarched linens. Your home linens will be softer than those used in the hospital where so much disinfectant is used. I suggest trying 100 percent cotton bedding because it absorbs perspiration well. However, you will have to use a fabric softener to keep it soft. Some patients like satin bedding, and particularly a satin pillow case is very comfortable.

The bedding must be kept dry and free of wrinkles and crumbs. Crumbs, wrinkles, and wetness destroy the patient's skin. It is practically impossible to heal bedsores in weakened cancer patients.

Linen can be changed while the patient remains in bed by rolling the patient to one side of the bed while changing the linen on the other side. Roll the patient onto the clean linen, walk to the other side of the bed, and finish exchanging the linen.

Some equipment to make the patient more comfortable may be readily available in your home. A large piece of paneling, pegboard, or pressed wood can be slipped under the mattress to make it more firm. An ordinary mattress may serve well for someone there for eight hours, but all-day bed rest requires a firmer mattress. Some people find a water bed or air mattress on top of a regular mattress provides better support by distributing the body pressure over a wider area to avoid bedsores. I find most people prefer remaining on the kind of mattress they have known their whole life, rather than switching to a waterbed when ill.

Extra pillows are a must so the patient can be propped into various positions. Also handy is a cool air vaporizer to provide moisture to a patient not assimilating liquids. Many cancer patients prefer the room cooler, especially if they start to run a fever due to bodily toxins. Adjust the temperature according to the patient's wishes.

Much of the equipment you need to care for a cancer patient is either already at home or easily rented. The only elaborate equipment you need to rent are the pumps or oxygen. Make sure the company will provide round-the-clock home service.

If You Are Employed

Home care can be managed even if the main caretakers are employed. You just have to make some plans.

My mother worked for many years and enjoyed her job. When Dad was sick at home during the first few months of his confinement, he was able to take care of himself. Later it became increasingly difficult for him to manage. When he became less mobile, he could not get himself to the kitchen or the bathroom. He was afraid of being stranded in the house in case of fire or other emergency. He never mastered the skill of giving himself shots, so someone had to be around to assist him when he had a bout of pain. Right after a heavy injection of narcotics, he could not read or interest himself in music or television, so time passed slowly for · him when he was alone.

Mother wanted to continue working for many reasons. She found that contact with people who were not sick provided some relief from round-the-clock nursing demands. Her friends provided some emotional support. Also, her job brought some financial security. Since she did not know how much time off she could get, she worked as long as Dad could manage by himself. When he needed full-time help, she stayed at home.

Other people I talked to wanted to keep their jobs for many of the same reasons. They fear losing their position by taking off too much time or they do not want to jeopardize their retirement or other benefits. The emotional benefits of an outside job cannot be underestimated. Most people have some fun at work with friends on the job. Doing the job makes the worker feel fulfilled. During the emotionally taxing times of losing a loved one to cancer, a job is a way of taking care of yourself. After the death, the job may be one of the constant contacts with people for the person left behind.

If you need to work and like to work, stay on the job. Home care can still be provided. You just have to make some plans. One of the plans that must be made is to hire someone to be with the patient when you are at work. Licensed practical nurses can handle the care for most cancer patients, and they are less expensive than hiring a registered nurse. Also, people who have worked as aides in a hospital can probably do the work you were doing at home once you train them in the routine.

Several sources are available for finding a nurse. Agencies can supply a nurse to fit your specifications. Advertising in the newspaper will bring applicants from whom you can make a choice. Another good source is a personal referral from an acquaintance who works in a hospital or doctor's office.

Several criteria must be considered for choosing a nurse. First, can he or she do the job? If the patient is large and must be moved, the nurse must be skilled in the principles of moving. One way to determine this is to ask the applicant to move the patient from the bed to the wheelchair during the interview. Not only will this show you if the applicant can do the job, but you also have the opportunity to observe the worker's attitude toward the patient. Did the applicant smile at the patient and speak to him gently before initiating the move? Did the applicant ask how the patient was feeling and conduct a conversation?

Checking references is another helpful source of information. Was the nurse reliable in coming to work every day as planned? Did she stay with the patient through to the end even when the going got rough? Was the nurse tidy and were proper nursing routines followed?

One of the most important sources of information is just how you and the patient feel about the nurse. The patient must have someone he feels comfortable being with. You can tell if their personalities clash. Did the patient smile or joke with the nurse on the interview when they were first introduced? If the nurse tells you that she is repelled by hopeless cases, I would look for someone else.

My father's insurance company paid for home nursing. We found there were enough of us around the house to manage during the days. But at night, we were tired and welcomed the extra help so we could all rest. One of us stayed up late with the nurse, another one of us got up early, so there were only a couple of hours that Dad did not have family immediately in his room. We were always available in the surrounding rooms, however.

If you work, you will need someone during the day when you are gone to stay with the patient. Hopefully, the patient will sleep through the night so you can get your rest. It is only at the very end when someone will have to sit next to the patient's bed round-the-clock. This is the time to take time off work so you can share the patient's last days. Some families like a four-hour nurse from late afternoon through the dinner hour so the needs of young children can be met for their dinners, homework, and bedtime routines.

One family I know hired a nurse for four hours during the afternoon. During the rest of the day one of the three college students in the family was available to help. They advertized and found an R.N. who was willing to come if she could bring her baby with her. The R.N. was cheerful, competent, and glad to have a part-time job where she did not have to be away from her baby. She charged less than agencies who must pay the nurse and their administrators. Agencies are reluctant to place people in less than eight hour shifts. The nurse was able to manage both the baby and the patient. The baby napped or played in the playpen she set up. When both the baby and the patient were awake, they entertained each other. Because this arrangement was so convenient for her, the R.N. remained on the job through to the end doing extra weekend duty as the family needed.

Hiring help has its problems. Some nurses will take the job and stay only a week without telling you they have another job waiting. It is discouraging to train someone only to have them quit. It is not unusual for family members to feel some jealousy when a nurse replaces them and does their job well. Patients perk up for the nurse and try to be pleasant. A few patients will be unusually gruff and drive nurses away. The family members feel justifiably angry because of the extra burden of continually having to find more help only to have a surly patient run them off. In this case, talk to the patient about a compromise between your needs to work and the patient's needs to have you constantly around.

Keeping Medical Records

Some doctors want medical records kept on the patient. Find out if the doctor wants them and if he or she has a form you can use to keep track. Usually there are two kinds of records the doctor wants: liquids in and out, and time and amount of pain medication.

Liquids in and out is important information because it helps the doctor judge how the kidneys are working. If the kidneys need help, the doctor wants advance notice because it takes time for his intervention to make a difference. Patients who retain liquid may become uncomfortably distended. If the patient becomes obstructed in his intestines, the doctor has to decide whether to put in a nasal-gastric tube to take out all liquids from the stomach or to try to remove the obstruction. One sign of uremic poisoning is decreased urine output. To know if what is coming out is adequate in amount, the doctor must know what is going in. Thus, you must keep records of all drinks, ice and any other liquid the patient takes by mouth and any liquid going in by other means such as an IV or an N-G. Output is primarily a measure of the amount of urine, but it also includes vomit.

Most doctors record in the metric system. You can buy an ordinary cc measure and pour all liquids in it for accurate metric measures. You can also get charts that convert ordinary household measures such as cups into metrics.

If metrics are too cumbersome or foreign to you, ask your doctor if you could please keep all measures in terms of cups, quarter-cups, measures you are familiar with.

We were keeping records on my father to make sure he did not become bloated. With an intestinal obstruction, he became very uncomfortable when liquids backed up, making him distended. It was very tedious to record everything he ate — each sip of water, half a popsicle, teaspoon of sherbert. Sometimes it was difficult to estimate how much he actually ate and how much remained in the cup. At the very end of his life, we abandoned the measures. He had a nasal-gastric tube, which extracted everything he ate. Since he had no IV, liquids were not given any way but mouth. Instead we watched carefully when we gave him drinks to see that everything came up immediately in the tube. The tube continually extracted some small amounts of liquid anyway, which were the stomach juices his body produced. As long as something was coming up the tube all the time, we were content that the N-G was doing its job properly.

The shot record is very necessary for the caretakers, patient, and doctor, so keep it meticulously. When a doctor gives you narcotics such as morphine to use at home, he or she is showing a lot of trust in your judgment. Morphine is typically given only in hospitals. It is an addictive and controlled substance, which means that you have to account for all you use and return the unused portions. Morphine is also dangerous. If too much is given to a terminal patient, it can damage the liver. Since pain medication must be metabolized by the liver before the body can use it, a damaged liver would mean that no pain medication could work. A patient with a severely damaged liver might still live, and all that time nothing would work for diminishing the pain because no medication would be metabolized.

Time passes differently when one is nursing a patient. Sometimes at night I would doze by Dad's side and lose track of time. When Dad requested an injection, I would check the chart and find out to my surprise that three hours had passed since the last shot. Other times it seemed to me that hours had passed when only minutes had. If I relied on my remembering how much time passed since the last injection, I am sure my estimates would be highly inaccurate.

A patient's requests for injections cannot be relied on to come consistently on time. If the patient is upset, he tends to ask for too many injections. When a patient is active, distracted, or preoccupied, he may go too long between shots and then become restless. If you wait too long between injections, you end up giving larger doses than you would ordinarily have to inject.

Keeping accurate shot records is a good idea. Record the time you give the shot and its location on the body. That way you will not give shots on top of each other. This will give the patient's skin an opportunity to recover. The hard shot lumps disappear when given time.

The shot record may look like the following:

SHOT RECORD FOR MORPHINE

Dosage: Quarter gram
Date, Time: Tuesday, January 17, 8:15 am
Location: Upper right thigh
Time since last shot: 3 hours

Keep a new sheet for each day. The sheet may be kept on a clipboard close to the medication so that the records can be filled out at the same time medication is given.

It is important to fill out the shot record immediately. With several people helping, it is easy to mix up who has done what when.

Some people keep daily logs of how the patient feels and any unusual physical changes. They record time of seizures, how good speech was, how far the patient walked, and any other information they judge to be relevant.

There are many uses for such a medical log. If the patient is receiving chemotherapy to cure or retard the disease, a medical log records any side effects that occur. When the doctor asks, "How is she doing?", you can tell with greater objectivity which specific changes have happened. Sometimes a pattern will emerge. Perhaps the doctor can diagnose the progress of the brain tumor from a description of the patient's behavior over a two-week period.

Another reason for keeping a medical log is to help you keep an objective view of the patient. The log forces you to look at the symptoms and the medical progress of the disease. This keeps you from slipping back into a denial pattern.

Keep the log just like you would keep a diary. Each day record your entry with as much description as you can: date, time, amount, color, quality. Describe carefully what you see. Take your log with you each time you visit the doctor so you can share accurate information. Jot down questions you want to ask the doctor as they occur to you or else the questions will be forgotten.

Keeping records for the doctor is an important part of your job. Keeping records for yourself — to clear your perceptions, to make a pattern out of symptoms, to record questions — gives the task more intrinsic appeal.

Chapter 3

MANAGING PAIN

F OR centuries, cancer carried the reputation of a pain causer. In the past, few pain killing medications were available, and pain was not as understood in its physical and psychological aspects as it is today. Modern medicine can manage well the physical aspects of pain.

For the second aspect of pain, the psychological side, physicians have little to offer. Typically, while the shots are working on the physical cause of pain, the fear and dread of the emotional side of pain ravage on.

Many variables enter into the perception of pain. The very expectation of pain can make the cancer patient more sensitive and may increase his or her response to pain stimuli.

Some personalities are more sensitive to pain. Research indicates that a darker skinned person will experience less pain than a fair skinned one, given the same pain stimulus. Whenever we are depressed or introspective, our responses to pain are heightened. Contrast this with a competitive game situation where a slight injury often goes unnoticed, since attention is turned outward. Most cancer patients are at times depressed and become increasingly introverted. It is not surprising that they grow increasingly sensitive to pain stimulation.

Pain differs if it is acute or chronic. Acute pain is usually sharp, strong, and transitory. It comes and goes, giving the person a chance to rest. Chronic pain is usually a dull pain present all the time. Chronic pain is harder to bear because it wears a person down. Both acute and chronic pain respond to pain medication and to diversionary techniques, described later in this chapter.

Patients tend to report more pain in the hospital than at home. In a hospital, a person is more tense and anxious. Anxiety heightens awareness of pain. Also, hospitalized cancer patients are often depressed and have a lot of time to think of their condition. There are a few diversions in the hospital. White bed, white walls. Time passes slowly. There is little to do. Heavily sedated, most people cannot read or bear to watch television. No wonder people with terminal illnesses who spend their last days in the hospital report a lot of pain. How hard it is for family members to sit in a hospital room with a person they love who is in pain and not be able to help.

Cancer is associated with severe pain in everyone's mind. When a person's cancer is diagnosed, two thoughts come to mind: cancer kills and cancer is painful. The second assertion is evidence for the first. Every time the cancer patient had a strong pain in the past, the doctor discovered bad news — the cancer had spread. Another organ was involved. Even a little pain becomes frightening because of what it means. A little pain over a long period wears a person down and becomes harder to bear than a stronger but short-lived pain. The future is bleak because all the patient has to look forward to is more pain and a weakening of his body.

Pain medication has little to offer for relief from the psychological aspects of pain. In a hospital, there is nothing to look at, no one to talk to except occasional guests, nothing to do but suffer until it is time for the next shot. The emotional causes of pain build up as the patient becomes increasingly less able to do for himself and more afraid of abandonment.

Management of pain is one of the most important reasons for dying at home. On the physical side, all the injections given at the hospital can be given at home. For the emotional aspects of pain, only family members and friends can help.

Everyone in my family mastered the injection technique in about ten minutes and became quite proficient at giving shots with practice. Dad preferred our efforts to the professional efforts of the nurses. Nurses told him the shot would not hurt. We told him we would try to be gentle. Please do not get me wrong; nurses were more skilled than us, but their attitude was different. We truly cared about every little intrusion on Dad's body.

All narcotics given to kill pain are available by prescription and can be administered at home with the approval of your physician. The doctor's nurse will tell you how often the shots can be given. You must account for the narcotics you use. The cost is about $5 per day, and you should have no problem keeping what is needed on hand and returning what is left over.

For the emotional aspects of pain, nurses are not the answer. Someone who cares is. A single nurse is responsible for ten to twenty patients. How does she care for all of them at the same time? Simple. She comes in only for the routine maintenance and physical aspects of nursing: giving medication, changing bandages, checking equipment, changing IV bottles. It is impossible for the nurse to attend to the various emotional needs of all her patients.

So if you ask yourself, who is providing the emotional care a dying person needs so desperately, the answer is no one probably, unless you are willing to do it.

Diversionary Techniques

The key to pain that medication cannot alleviate is to provide a stimulus to compete with the pain stimulus. Of the various stimuli available, touching is a good stimulus to obliterate pain. Just holding hands or rubbing the patient's arm works beautifully. Backrubs are excellent. The stronger the pain, the stronger the backrub needed. Rubbing the chest or legs is also good. A cool cloth on the forehead brings relief. The trick is to give the patient something to think about or feel besides pain and to provide reassurance that the patient does not have to face the pain alone.

It sounds surprising that touching can compete with narcotics. Ask any cancer or geriatric nurse. She will tell you how amazing it is when physical contact is made. Pain is lessened or goes away almost completely. Sometimes the patient thinks he had been given a shot when all that had been done was to rub him down.

The natural childbirth movement uses this principle. Fear increases pain. A muscle spasm without fear is just a muscle spasm, not excruciating discomfort. In natural childbirth, the mother learns to relax with contractions and take her mind off pain by performing breathing exercises. Relaxation enables women to go through childbirth without pain medication or with much less than mothers who are not relaxed. Mothers trained in natural childbirth techniques generally tend to remember the birth process as a wonderful experience, while anesthesized mothers either remember nothing or have some pain memories.

Pain killers are only partially effective for labor pains, while the mother trained in natural childbirth perceives them as spasms that she can control. Much of cancer pain is of the spasm type, which makes it respond to the same techniques as those used in natural childbirth. Relaxation, deep breathing during moderate pain, and pant-blow breathing during strong pain all help. The mental attitude of being in control, pulling one's consciousness above and away from the pain also helps.

Another technique of natural childbirth called "effleurage" works well with cancer pain. Effleurage is gentle massage of the abdomen with the fingers slightly rotating in big circles. Both hands meet and come up the center of the abdomen, part, and go down the sides. Effleurage provides a pleasant stimulus to compete with abdominal pain. With pain at other sites of the body, effleurage helps keep the patient relaxed while providing something for him to do with his hands. The mind must be concentrating on deep rhythmic breathing and moving away from the pain to thoughts of a better time. Mind trips, which I explain later, are helpful at this point.

Massaging gives the patient something else to feel besides pain. He or she is tired of feeling pain and welcomes another stimulus. Massaging provides a soothing relaxation from pain. The gentle touch reassures the patient you are present, you are trying to help, and you will not leave. You presence is attested to by touch during moments the patient's eyes are out of focus due to pain medication or consciousness that slips in and out. By being present to massage, you are also available to listen to the patient's fears, which will tend to revolve around three issues: fear of pain, abandonment, and dying. Some studies cite a fourth fear, suffocation.

Touching was the main way my family made contact with my father during the last week of his life when he was dissociating himself from his body and his surroundings. He conversed very little. All communication had to come from touch. JoAnn, the youngest daughter, was having a hard time reconciling herself to Dad's imminent death, so she massaged his back rather than talk. Soon she discovered Dad could carefully get up, sit on the edge of a chair, bend over forward, and rest his head on a pillow on the bed. She kneaded his tight neck and shoulder muscles, overworked from being propped up in the bed. JoAnn did not have to say anything; she knew she did something important for Dad.

It is not always necessary to think in terms of backrubs, although they are a good way to begin. A good practice is to rub the patient's thigh or upper arm where the shot is to be given. It serves not only to comfort both you and the patient but also to keep the skin in good tone, since rubbing promotes good circulation.

It was very interesting to us to see how Dad's perception of pain changed depending on what we were doing. In the hospital Dad would have spasms of pain and would call for a shot. Waiting until it came was hard for him and us. We would tense up, hold his hand, fight back tears, and wait feeling anguished if he had to suffer long. The most active part we took at first was looking for a nurse if his call light was not answered. Soon we began taking a more active role in this difficult situation. Dad would tell us of his pain, and we would go into action. We rolled him over, massaged his back, and applied cool compresses. The position of the bed was changed to relieve any cramped organs and promote circulation. We always talked in low, gentle, rhythmic tones. By the time the shot came, he was usually comfortable. At home Dad had less pain. He was more relaxed as we all were knowing pain medication was immediately available. But when he had pain, he no longer called for a shot. He just alerted us. Right away two of us began working on him, rubbing, bathing or talking. If two hours had passed since his last injection, another was administered. Often just the massaging made him think an injection had been given.

It is important to remember that pain medication works best to ward off pain not yet present rather than to get rid of a serious pain. It is better to give injections by the clock even if the patient feels all right rather than wait too long and then have the injection handle only part of the pain. Remember, pain is harder to diminish than to keep away completely. If you wait too long to give an injection and give the pain time to build up, it will be harder to eradicate. A good operating rule is that the patient can have a shot as often as every two hours if he wishes, but do not let him go longer than four hours between injections unless the physician advises otherwise.

Anything that provides a diversion from the pain is enhancing the effect of pain medication. Eating, drinking, mouthwash, relaxation, music in headphones, alcohol sponge bath, mints, a walk outdoors in the wheelchair, being turned to a new position, all serve as diversions to pain, so do not underestimate their importance. They do not replace pain killing medication; they augment the influence of the medication, helping until it starts to work and helping it work better.

Diversionary techniques combat both causes of pain. On the physical side, they reduce the tension and muscle cramps that contribute to pain. On the emotional side, the techniques reassure the patient, reducing his fears that you will not help him when the going gets rough.

Cognitive Behavioral Approaches to Pain Management

Research has shown that all pain has a cognitive component. This means that the way we think about pain and respond to it emotionally will influence how bad it feels. Work with patients with chronic pain that has persisted over six months indicates that mind control and relaxation can overcome pain that narcotics cannot touch.

While there are numerous behavioral techniques that will be presented for the patient to try, all require a deep relaxation. The patient should practice achieving deep relaxation at least twice a day until an almost trancelike state can be obtained. Try following this procedure:

1. Tense the muscles in the feet and hold them tense for ten seconds. Then release the muscles and feel the relaxation flow in. Try to make the rest of the body feel as relaxed as the feet.

2. Keeping the feet and the body above the knees relaxed, tense the calves of the legs and hold it tense for ten seconds before re-

leasing. Try to achieve a deep relaxation below the knees as though the legs were buried in warm sand. Think pleasant thoughts or visualize a relaxing scene from nature while doing the relaxation exercise.

3. Tense the thighs, hold for ten seconds, then relax for ten seconds.

4. Tense the buttocks while the rest of the body is relaxed. Hold for ten seconds and then release. Be conscious of the absence of tension while you visualize a clear mountain lake.

5. Pull the stomach back toward the backbone and hold for ten seconds. Then push it out and hold it extended for ten seconds before releasing the muscles. Many people carry tension in their stomach, so this part of the exercise may be repeated as many times as it takes for the stomach muscles to feel relaxed.

6. Keeping the rest of the body relaxed, tense the muscles in the hands, arms and shoulders. After holding it for ten seconds, release.

7. Tense every muscle in the face, grimacing, sticking out the tongue, tensing the neck muscles and pulling the scalp muscles by raising the eye brows. Hold this for ten seconds. Release and feel the relaxation flow down from the top of the head to meet with the rest of the body.

8. Mentally check the body for relaxation. Any part that is not relaxed should be tensed, held, and then released. Couple the feeling of calm with a pleasant scene and soothing thoughts.

Remember what you usually think of when you are in pain. Most people tense up and think something like, "I hurt; I have excruciating pain. I cannot stand it. The pain is going to kill me." The common elements in a typical response to pain are muscle tenseness and negative, fearful thoughts. Cognitive behavioral approaches to pain management achieve the reduction of pain sensation by changing both of those reactions.

The first thing to do when in pain is to relax. Start breathing deeply and slowly or perhaps panting or blowing if the pain is sharp. Then start to relax, either lying down flat or curled up.

The next step is called "thought stopping." The negative thoughts about how bad the pain is must be stopped. Some patients just say "Stop!" loudly when they notice themselves feeling afraid.

After the thoughts are stopped, there are various techniques that the patient can choose from. Some patients try a different technique each time; others find a routine that works for them and use it without variation. All techniques have been found to be helpful.

Relabeling the pain involves the patient calling the pain something else. Perhaps the patient will say, "My leg is cold" or "My back is numb." Maybe the knee is warm or the foot is pulsating, but no longer does the patient use the word "pain" in speech or thought.

Some patients find that centering on the pain helps diminish it so they will focus all of their attention on the pain area, even looking at it when possible. While focusing attention on the pain site, the patient repeats that the area is numb and makes coping statements such as "I can handle this" or "I know I can remain relaxed for the few minutes it takes to finish."

Other patients redirect their attention away from the pain area. They relax and focus on a relaxing scene. Some turn all of their attention on a real or imagined blank wall, visualizing each crevice and imperfection in detail. Some patients redirect their attention to a different part of the body. One helpful technique is to slap a part of the body not in pain, say a thigh, and concentrate on that feeling rather than the pain. Taking a warm, soothing bath or a cold, penetrating shower are variations on the same theme.

Try various techniques until one seems to work routinely. Remember that the keys are relaxation, stopping negative thoughts, reprogramming thoughts to positive ones of being able to cope, and directing attention.

Mind Trips

A strategy that might be used to take the patient's mind off his discomfort is called taking a mind trip. A mind trip is simply returning by memory to a place both of you remember fondly by constructing every single detail about the place.

Describe your mind trip in the present tense, relating events, sights, smells, and feelings as though it were really happening at the current moment. Use a low, melodious tone and ask the patient no questions. A mind trip is not a conversation, it is a monologue. The patient floats away on the mind trip, so to speak. By rendering the patient to a dreamy state, pain medication is conductive to this visit to a more pleasant time in the past.

You will find it easy to imagine going step-by-step through the journey. Then you will not have to think ahead to what you will find but instead you will discover details you thought were forgotten as you perhaps romped through waist high snow building a snowman in the. front yard or drove the familiar route to your grandparent's house.

Our first mind trip was to a park near where my father grew up. It was the location of many family outings. I started our mind trip by loading up the car with the aromatic foods for our picnic. We drove to the park over scenic roads both Dad and I knew well. As we neared the park we saw Lake Nokomis. I described the lake in detail: how it looked like a large mirror glistening with sunlight and surrounded by lush green trees. Multicolored sailboats skimmed across the water, their bright colors reflected on the surface of the lake like flags fluttering in a high wind. At this point my father said with his eyes closed, "Look at all the gulls flying by shore." I replied that today there were more birds than I had ever seen before. He agreed.

The pain medication produces a surreal state where the patient can easily float in and out of various stages of consciousness. This contributes to the success of the mind trips. More important, mind trips provide a vehicle the patient can use to escape from the sometimes dreary discomforting existence of sickness to happier times. The pain remains in the sick world.

Sometimes the patient will ask for a mind trip back to a place you have never seen, such as his Army days or his childhood. For these trips describe universally present impressions such as clouds, trees and gentle breezes. Center on something in your own experience that must have been present then. You can always talk about the different shapes of billowing white clouds against a clear blue sky, a brilliant sunset, or the cool sliver of a moon against a black crisp sky.

A mind trip is a reconstruction of a pleasant time. It is important to speak calmly, softly, and happily about these good times. You are not speaking with regret. You are sharing your memory bank of fond times together, times you are grateful to have had once and now you can have them again. By speaking softly and melodically, you create almost a hypnotic effect that promotes deep relaxation and greatly alleviates pain. This is yet another reason for caring for your loved one. No nurse has the shared memories you have, nor can a nurse usually create the trust it takes to go along on a mind trip.

When the pain or weariness became too much to bear, Dad would say, "Let's leave it." So we left the dreary world of shots and escaped from a diseased body to a much better time. Dad relaxed, the lines in his face disappearing as we visited hand-in-hand the peaceful days of the past. On our picnic trip we reached the park and saw that the rest of the family had arrived. Dad recognized his mother, who had died ten years earlier, also of cancer. He brought this theme up later and then I realized its psychological importance.

The memories of a lifetime provide an unlimited supply of itineraries. Mind trips also serve the function of showing the patient that his or her life was not lived in vain. Many moments were lived fully.

Mind trips open the door to communication in situations when you have run out of things to say. Your vast wealth of shared experiences and happy memories give you something to say that is not associated with sickness and discomfort. It gets tiring to continue to say, "Are you in pain? Do you want a drink? Shall I roll the bed up?" A mind trip also shows that the good times are not forgotten or contaminated by these difficult times. The many happy, loving moments will live on.

Mind trips also provide a way for the patient to speak about dying in a symbolic way that is less threatening than talking about dying directly.

The symbolism of dying becomes more pronounced as time passes. In our mind trips, Dad always wanted two people present, my mother and his mother. I think he wanted my mother present because it was hard for him to think about leaving his wife. He wanted his mother present because she represented where he was going, since she had died previously. Dad pictured himself as walking with our family and having to go off a long way to get to his mother. I incorporated this theme in one of our mind trips to help him work through this transition, which was so difficult for him. I told him that his mother was far off in the distance on a grassy hill, next to a tall oak tree. My mother and their children were walking with him toward her. At this point, Dad interrupted me saying he had a fence to climb because it was in the way, but he did not know how to do it. I asked him if he was afraid to climb it and he said he was. I assumed this meant he was afraid of the mystery of death, not knowing how to die or what it would be like. I said we would take him to one side of the fence and his mother would take his hand and help him climb to the other side. He would never be alone; we would turn him over to her.

This particular mind trip brought my father great peace. He had been unable to speak about his fears of dying, but he obviously worried about what it would be like. Our mind trip was like a practice run. Many times the same theme came up, and for Dad there was always a fence he had to climb.

With other patients I notice the symbolism, though slightly different, is often present. They may have a mountain or a hill to climb, a long road to walk, a trip to take, or a river to cross. If there is some obstacle to their progress, the symbolism of death may be indicated. The patients are working through the problem of what their own death will be like. With a mind trip you provide the patient with someone who understands the symbolism. You let the patient go over and over the problem until the patient feels comfortable enough about it to consider it finished. The assistance you can provide with a mind trip is to help the patient to come up with an acceptable image of what death will be like.

For Dad, I told him we would transfer him from our care to the loving care of his mother. When I told him we would bring a step stool he could use to get over the fence, I was symbolically releasing him. He knew we wanted him to be able to go easily when the time came.

Alleviating Pain by Medication

Medications to counteract pain can be given by mouth, injection, or IV. Steriods counteract pain by relieving inflammation, antibiotics by ridding infections, and analgesics by modifying the perceptions of pain or the reaction to the sensation of pain. Analgesics may be non-narcotic such as aspirin or narcotic such as the opiate morphine. In general, narcotics are stronger and more effective for intense pain than non-narcotic analgesics. However, narcotics have drawbacks such as making the patient dependent on them in ever-increasing dosages if they are used over a long time. Although some analgesics are specific for a certain type of pain, most are nonspecific. Aspirin will work on a headache or a toothache. Thus, analgesics can usually be used interchangeably for various types of pain.

That narcotics make a cancer patient dependent on them is not a major concern for the terminal cancer patient. Dependence means that the patient will manifest physical withdrawal symptoms when deprived of the drug. These commonly entail restlessness but may also include fever, runny nose, nausea, and muscle cramps. Cancer patients are seldom taken off pain medication, so these symptoms are not a problem. Typically, the cancer patient is put on narcotics at the end of his or her life and stays on them for the time remaining.

Cancer patients generally do not exhibit any of the signs known as drug addiction, which is different from drug dependence. Addiction is abuse of a drug. Dependence is a legitimate need and use for a drug. There is no drug that will reduce or eliminate intense pain without resulting in some dependence.

The main responsibility of the physician is to monitor the amount of pain medication given to avoid too high a tolerance for the drug. More and more of the narcotic is needed to do the same job, but the body cannot tolerate so much of the drug. The liver, in particular, can be damaged by high doses of narcotics. The physician must keep the patient on a long-term drug plan where the least potent drug is used at first with the doses kept at the smallest amount that will do the job. Doses are slowly increased until they are so large that the patient must be switched to another, more potent drug. Again doses in the new drug are as 'small as possible. The physician has to gauge how long the patient will live to make sure a drug in a dose the body can tolerate will handle all the pain until the patient dies.

Drug addiction is not the concern with cancer patients as drug tolerance is. Tolerance means that more and more of a drug must be administered to produce the same effect even though the pain level remains constant. Often the problem is compounded by the fact that the pain is getting worse while the effect of the initial level of the drug is becoming less effective.

When morphine is given twice a day, tolerance begins to develop in about ten days. Usually, morphine is given more often than twice a day. If the pain gets worse, more morphine is needed, and the result is often less effective. Tolerance can be eliminated if the patient is not given the drug for a week or two. However, this is not practical for a patient with continuous pain. Different drugs are alternated when possible, with morphine reserved for the last part of life. Demerol® and other analgesics are used as long as possible. When a patient is switched to morphine, it is usually with the thought that it will serve him until he or she dies.

The goal is for the patient to be comfortable, yet aware and responsive. If the patient is continually in a lot of pain, the doctor should be notified so the drugs given can be reevaluated. The patient should not be overmedicated. The diversionary techniques for pain management should be used instead of narcotics whenever possible. This way you are ensuring that the narcotics will be effective throughout the patient's life.

My father was told about his terminal cancer seven months before he died. At first he took pain pills only occasionally. A few weeks later he was taking them rather regularly. Sometimes the pills either would not handle the pain spasms or would work too slowly. Then he received pain medication given by injection at home as needed. He would go many days without any medication. Then he would have a bad night and need one or more shots. If the pain was intense and continued for some time, the doctor would hospitalize him for a couple of days until the cause of the pain had been handled. Then he could go home and the routine continued: shots as needed, extreme pain that could not be handled at home, hospitalization and then back home. This went on for six months until the pain could no longer be eradicated in the hospital. Dad was switched to morphine, on which he was fairly comfortable, and the final phase of his life began. Throughout this entire period, diversionary techniques were extremely important.

In a study of the drugs administered to 100 terminal cancer patients of all adult ages in a private hospital, researchers found a pattern similar to the one of my father. Most patients start with pain killers such as Darvon® or codeine, which are given until about a month before death. Then the patient is given Demerol, which is the most frequently used narcotic. Demerol is used at a steady and high level until close to death, when most patients are switched to morphine.

Other medicines may be given with the pain medications. Seconal® is a sleeping pill, which some patients are told to use as needed. Chlorpromazine is an anti-nausea medicine, which also makes other pain medications work better. By itself chlorpromazine does not relieve pain; it just makes the other drug more effective. It also relaxes the patient. When tenseness goes, the pain goes, which is the principle of the diversionary techniques.

The syringes to inject Demerol are disposable. Plastipak® or Jelco® are both good and cheap. There is nothing to sterilize because the whole syringe comes put together and sterile in a pre-packaged form, which is used, and discarded. Demerol needles are long because the drug must be injected into the muscle. Break off the needle from the syringe after use so that a child would not be tempted to play doctor with it if found in the garbage.

Morphine is injected with a short needle right under the skin. The Tubex® holder of the glass cartridge with the drug inside is reusable. The cartridge with its sterile needle is screwed into the Tubex, used, and discarded after the needle is broken off for safety.

How to Give Shots

Learning how to give shots is easy. With Demerol, which is what you will probably start with, it is especially easy because the syringe is all put together for you. The Tubex is really no problem either. The device is opened and the cartridge is slipped in. The cartridge is screwed to the right to secure it in the Tubex. Then the plunger is closed over the cartridge and screwed tight. You pull back on the plunger and then start to depress it slowly until all the air is out of the cartridge.

The next task is to choose a place on the patient's body to put the shot. There are many possible sites: the upper arm, the upper front and upper back thigh, and the hip. Feel the site with your finger. If you find a hard lump, it means a shot was given there before and you should find another place. Record the location of each shot on the shot record to avoid overusing the convenient locations such as the upper arm.

Once you decide on a location, swab it down with alcohol. The prepackaged swabs are convenient and inexpensive. Each comes in a foil wrapper so it is always sterile. After swabbing, take a big pinch of skin and insert the needle. There are style differences in method of insertion. The "plungers" push the needle in quickly to get the injection over with. The "wigglers" move the needle back and forth until it pierces the skin. I cannot make a case for one style over the other even though I am a modified wiggler; you will develop your own style, the one you feel is best.

When the needle is inserted all the way, draw it back a little before you begin depressing the plunger. Very infrequently you will see a little blood indicating that the needle has hit a small blood vessel. You must pull the needle out, swab another location and give the shot elsewhere.

Usually there will be no blood when you pull back so you can depress the plunger. Depress it slowly to avoid lumps. Do not depress too slowly — it should take no longer than 3 seconds to put the medicine in the patient. Then pull out the needle and reswab the area. Break the needle and dispose of it and the cartridge. Reinsert a new cartridge so everything is ready for an emergency. Do not remove the rubber tip covering the needle until you are ready to put the needle into the patient because the tip keeps the needle sterile.

If you give a shot because the patient requests one for pain, the patient will still have pain for a few moments after the injection is given. Rather than let the patient sit and suffer, give a backrub during the time it takes the medicine to work. This will take the patient's mind off the pain, relax his or her muscles, which have tensed in response to the pain and are intensifying it. The patient may well relax so much that he or she will drift off to sleep.

Shots present a psychological barrier to some people. It would help to grow up with a diabetic who took insulin shots daily, but not everyone has had the experience nor is it necessary for getting over the fear of giving shots. If you are around someone who takes shots, you lose that reluctance to give them yourself. Much of the fear of shots is a carryover from childhood. In fact, giving or getting a shot is not so bad. For cancer patients shots usually have a positive connotation because of the relief the pain medication brings.

We viewed giving the shot as an act of love. When it was shot time, everyone wanted to give the injection to help Dad, so we had to take turns. Dad never minded that we amateurs practiced on him. He said we were more gentle than the nurses. Also, not having to wait when he wanted a shot was a real advantage.

Being able to give injections at home is what frees you from being forced to leave the patient in the hospital. The freedom to give pain medicine when the patient needs it relieves the fears the patient has about suffering alone in a hospital room with no one to help.

A legitimate reason to give pain medication is to relieve physical discomfort. An illegitimate reason to give pain medication is to knock out a patient who is angry, depressed or complaining. The normal reaction for the cancer patient is to feel angry or afraid about his predicament. He may be irritable with his family, demanding something and then rejecting it when it comes. Or the patient may cry profusely. Remember that anger and sadness are all normal, natural and predictable responses to cancer. They are necessary parts of the process of working toward acceptance. If they do not happen, the patient will probably not reach the stage of peace. I do not feel that anger or depression are valid reasons for putting the patient on emotional tranquilizers such as Valium®, Librium®, Vistaril®, Thorazine®, Mellaril®, or Stelazine®. Some patients appreciate taking a tranquilizer occasionally or for some short period of time, but the best thing psychologically for the patient is to express and work through these feelings. It is better to resolve them than to disguise them.

The problem with the major tranquilizers is that they render the patient unable to express his fears. Even though the patient looks improved, the fears and anger are still there and will return in full force when the tranquilizer wears off. Precious time has been wasted, and the work toward acceptance remains. It has been my experience that patients are tranquilized because their families cannot accept the illness. It may take some professional counseling to remedy this situation.

Radiotherapy

Besides pain medication, some tumors respond to radiotherapy to reduce pain. Undesirable side effects of radiation are seldom seen, since a small dose is usually given. Long-term effects of radiation are not a concern if the cancer is terminal.

Radiotherapy will not work in all cases. For some cancers, the dose required to reduce pain is as large as the dose used to try to burn out the tumor, so side effects would be felt. The decision to try radiotherapy to relieve pain is a highly individual one.

Usually radiotherapy is effective for pain reduction in those cases where the pain is localized. It is generally not effective when pain is all over, such as emanating from the whole abdomen.

Head and neck cancers often respond reasonably well to moderate doses of radiotherapy. For instance, with a large tumor mass in the oral cavity, patients often have pain behind the mouth and ear. With advanced, localized lesions, some patients who were not radiated as part of their treatment reported benefit from high dosages of radiotherapy — 5,000 rads total dose given over a seven-week period. Split-dosage radiotherapy, where the patient has two rest periods lasting two to four weeks in the midst of treatment, is often beneficial because it gives patients time to recover and perhaps avoid the side effects that may occur from a single series of daily treatments.

The severe headache associated with intracranial tumors or the pounding headache from a superior vena cava obstruction lung cancer may respond to irradiation of the brain. Pain from lung lesions that involve the brachial plexus usually does not respond to irradiation. However, pain from the rib or chest wall involvement associated with lung tumors may be reduced by radiotherapy. When lung or breast cancer has metastatic lesions in the thorax, pain can usually be significantly reduced by moderate doses of radiation. Metastases respond to smaller doses of irradiation than do primary tumors.

Breast cancer metastases generally respond well to radiation. Pain from soft-tissue involvement of the breast, usually accompanied by ulceration and bleeding, can be lessened with a rapid course of radiotherapy given in moderate doses. The same is true of osteolytic breast cancer metastases to pelvic bones. When radiotherapy is delivered to the involved area in doses of 2,500 to 4,000 rads in two to four weeks, about 80 percent of the patients can expect marked alleviation of pain. Over half of the patients experience relief from pain due to breast cancer metastases to bones of the extremities.

Cancer patients with abdominal problems are often helped by radiotherapy. In patients with gastrointestinal obstruction for whom diversionary bowel surgery is not possible and the pain cannot be controlled by medication, radiotherapy may provide relief in some cases. Patients with genitourinary obstruction from primary kidney or ureteral tumors or from lymph node or retroperitoneal cancer may obtain a reduction in pain when radiation beams can be properly focused on the involved areas. Usually some preliminary work must be done first. Laparotomy to assess the extent of the tumor and urinary diversion with a skin ureterostomy or ileal pouch must be completed first. Some patients may not want to undergo these procedures, or they may not be strong enough for them. The pros and cons can be discussed with the physician.

Chronic leukemia patients may have acute episodes of pain from splenomegaly or splenic infarctions. Rapid relief of pain can be achieved by small doses of radiation, 700 to 2,000 rads, in ten days to three weeks.

Radiation can reduce pain from many kinds of primary bone tumors. If selected sites can be identified and irradiated, pain can be reduced from the painful lesions in Ewing's sarcoma and multi-

ple myeloma. Less likely to respond to irradiation are osteo-
sarcomas and chondrosarcomas, although in the terminal stage,
one has nothing left to lose by trying.

If the pain comes from the pelvis, radiotherapy may offer
relief. Rectal tenesmus in unresectable rectal cancer may be
lessened with high doses of radiation. Radiation may also help
perineal recurrence of rectal cancer. In this kind of disease, even
small lesions cause great discomfort when the patient sits. When
bladder cancer has caused urinary tenesmus, implanting a number
of radioactive isotopes interstitially may give relief as will external
supervoltage irradiation. If the bladder is chronically infected,
urinary diversions may be required. If the patient has multiple
sites of pelvic intestinal obstruction, radiotherapy probably will
not help, but again if surgery is impossible, radiation might be
worth a try.

Painful lesions from other types of cancer that may respond to
radiation include metastatic lesions in the bones of the extremities from bronchogenci, prostatic, thyroid, or kidney cancers. Also
known to respond to irradiation are lesions from lymphomas and
osteoblastic metastases to the pelvis from prostate cancer. The
pain offshoots of esophageal cancer can be ultimately relieved
from irradiation although sometimes the pain increases right before it decreases.

If you seek help for the patient from various specialists, it is
important that you know the medical terminology for the kind of
cancer your loved one has. Where are the metastatic lesions
and what are they called? Ask your physician to write down the
medical terminology relating to your patient and carry the paper
with you. Then you can refer to it when doing things as diverse as
reading a technical article in the library to consulting with a specialist.

Chapter 4

FACILITATING COMMUNICATION

THE dying person and those around him or her go through many emotions regarding how they feel about themselves and the illness. Many of these feelings are difficult for the patient and the family, but they can be worked through. Successfully resolving the conflicts surrounding dying leads the terminal cancer patient and all involved to a feeling of peace about the situation and even of death. These feelings tend to follow a pattern.

Adjustment is a quiet time of almost no feeling. The wrenching pain and anguish of before dissipate. I do not want to fool you — the emotional pain is not replaced by happiness. Sometimes the anguish is supplanted by a numb feeling of emptiness. At other times there is more neutrality and plain acceptance than existential feelings of nothingness, but typically the result is tranquil.

The important thing is that the despair and hostility subside. Instead the patient feels that when and if death should come, he or she is ready to go. The family concedes that it is all right for the patient to leave. Then the family and the patient can work together to make the parting a loving one. The goals are to facilitate communication about dying, to ventilate negative feelings, and to resolve conflicts.

To be told one has terminal cancer results in a shock. The mind tries to protect the person from harsh reality by putting up shields, called defense mechanisms, to keep the person from collapsing under the tragic burden. These defense mechanisms cause reality to be viewed differently than the way it really is.

This distortion is initially helpful, since without it the person could not cope with the truth. In time, the defense mechanisms ease up or change, permitting more of reality to filter in, giving the person a chance to adjust.

Numerous professionals have investigated the process of dying. The patients and family members in my counseling groups tended to follow a common pattern of changing feelings, but wide individual variability between individuals still existed. The emphasis of this book is on helping people through the unpleasant aspects of adjusting to dying from terminal cancer. By resolving the main issues and problems, the patient has about his condition, some of the difficult stages of dying are either passed over completely or progressed through quickly. The way the patient adjusts to dying affects how the rest of the family feels.

The main factor that influences an onset of a particular type of a stage is the cancer patient's basic personality style. People who are driving, competitive types will exhibit similar behavior during their illness with the probable onset of the coping process in the searching phase. The prevailing reaction of depressed people will be probably deepening of the despair. Hostile people will continue to be angry and to blame others, persisting in their demands and at the same time rejecting efforts to help. These personality traits may both determine the onset of a phase type and may also overshadow or interact with the hypothesized phase the patient is thought to be in.

Some people may not resolve their conflict and may die feeling angry or depressed. You have to accept this as a possibility. Remember that if the patient has been angry his whole life, to be angry about dying may be a perfectly normal reaction on his part. That particular patient is dying just as he lived.

Following are some typical reactions to cancer, excerpted from case notes on some patients whose reactions followed the most common reactions of repression, hostility, searching, despair and finally, adjustment. Examples of what to say may give you an idea about the types of insight the patient needs to acquire to successfully resolve the conflict.

Shock Leading to Repression

Shock is the most usual initial reaction to hearing the bad news that the disease has progressed uncontrollably. The patient cannot believe the truth. Sometimes he will request duplicate lab tests. Another will find a new doctor. The shock or denial leads to repression, which is a defense mechanism protecting the patient from mental anguish. The emotions become numb. The patient feels nothing in order to keep himself from feeling too much and being overwhelmed.

The first phase is not necessarily a sad time. For some it is full of a sort of unrealistic hope based on a fantasy conception of the situation. Besides moments when the awesomeness of the situation momentarily overwhelms the patient, life goes on as usual.

One of my patients, Allan, a fifty-year-old man, went out of his way to keep his life on the same routine it had always followed. Al's wife reported he followed the clock exactly, leaving the house for work at precisely the time he was supposed to. Saturdays Al went to the golf course even if the weather would not permit golfing. The only thing Al did differently was that he stopped going to his doctor. As the disease started to weaken him, Al fought all the harder to keep to his routine as though his life depended on it. In a sense it did.

Because repression is not an accurate reality conception, other emotions are being held in check by it. For some people, maybe most, fear motivates the shock. For others, anger accompanies the shock. This is apparent when the patient denies the cancer by debasing the doctor who made the diagnosis. Given the underlying turmoil and protection of repression, it is generally best to allow the patient to come through this phase on his own. Repression serves the function of putting distance between the person and the diagnosis until the patient is ready emotionally to attend to that issue. Repression protects the patient from the shock of the truth.

Silence is one way to deal with repression. Since I choose not to tell a white lie to my patients, I cannot be an accomplice to the denial. I do not want to say something cruel, which is what the truth is at this point, so I say nothing. I hold the patient's hand or listen sympathetically and say, "It sure is hard sometimes, isn't it?" I set up the groundwork for later communication by being available and trying to help in any way possible. Initially, when a patient's denial is accepted, it gives him a chance to hear how his arguments sound. Soon the patient will question these arguments, and the stage is set for moving on to a more realistic appraisal of the situation. Some people, however, will not have enough remaining time to move past repression.

I was called in by an Intensive Care Unit physician to work with the family of a young woman, Ruth, who had sustained severe injuries in a car accident. She was expected to die in a matter of hours. The problem was that Ruth insisted on talking about the future at this time, and her family had difficulties accepting what they understood as wasting precious moments. When I listened to Ruth, it was obvious that she was making plans for her infant and her husband to follow when she was gone. She was talking about the preschool she would send her son to and the color she picked out for the house, as a way of leaving a verbal will or legacy. It was painful for this new mother to contemplate leaving her child and husband, but she also knew she may have to, so she spent her last moments thinking about their future and trying to make a final contribution to it.

Outside the ICU, I coached the family to listen and to go along with Ruth's denial. There was not enough time for Ruth to work through her anger at being cheated out of life so young or her depression at having to leave her loving family. There was not time for the family to work through all of their similar feelings. All we could do was use the last moments for loving listening and acceptance of what Ruth wanted to say. She died giving orders about the ideal babysitter, a matter of practical concern for her husband.

Most families find it easy to go along with a patient's repression because the patient says what the family wants to hear. Many cancer patients look normal and healthy for a long time. It is hard to believe the patient is terminally ill. It is easy to believe the patient will recover, since this is what everyone wants to believe.

With my father, the denial encompassed the whole family. He was told twice before that he would die soon, eight years and

seventeen years before the final diagnosis of terminal cancer. Since
he had beaten the rap twice, it was easy to believe he would get
by again and fool the doctors by outliving them. This time the
doctors said they were not completely sure it was cancer because
they could not safely biopsy the liver. The scans and the history
made them pretty sure without a biopsy. But the family preferred
to think otherwise.

The time to give a corrective response to a patient's denial
response is when the repression goes on for months and is hurting
the patient or his family. I start by making statements indicating
that I find it hard to accept the denial argument. I will say, "You
could be right, but I really do not think so."

One of my middle-aged patients, Danny, had steadfastly
denied the evidence of his lung cancer metastases. He had taken a
long-planned vacation in a motor home. I thought the trip was a
good idea because it would leave Danny and his wife with fond
memories to tide them over the hard times ahead. After the trip,
he suggested to help pay for the trip's costs by postponing the
payments of his insurance premiums. His wife had accepted the
cancer diagnosis and that she would have to raise their three
young children alone, but she was becoming highly irritated with
him for continuing with denial in the face of evidence to the
contrary up to the point of jeopardizing his family's future well-
being.

One evening the family sat down with Danny and told him
how they felt about the cancer. They did not wish to deny the
existence of cancer any longer, but of course they still held out
some hope he would live a long life. Mostly, they felt a need to
put their financial affairs in order so that in case something
happened to any of them, not just Danny, the others would not
have such a difficult time carrying on.

This scene took place in my office where the family had re-
hearsed what to say. Their remarks were as gentle as possible
without falling into the denial pattern.

Initially, Danny did not want the subject of cancer to be dis-
cussed at all. Later, he addressed the cancer issue. His reactions
were angry. He was angry at the doctors and blamed them for
their inability to cure the disease. Also, he was furious at the

tobacco industry for questioning the evidence about the relationship between lung cancer and cigarettes. Then he lashed out at the government for providing him with free cigarettes during the military service.

His wife quietly pointed out that anyone in the room could conceivably die in an hour. The point of the meeting was not that she wanted to profit from his death. She worried how the family could survive. She said, "I am worried about where to get grocery money to feed this brood of ours."

The children were in my waiting room playing rather loudly. Danny looked in their direction at the closed door. "Men have to provide for their families." he said. Among the things he wanted to provide for was a vacation next summer. This was a kind of denial response, again not allowing the presence of the cancer to hamper his plans. But also, it was a bargaining response: if I plan a vacation for next year, I will be around to go on it. He continued with planning of family affairs as though to say, "If I am the perfect husband and father, I will be granted a reprieve from this punishment."

The family worked well together on mutual plans for weeks. Then one of his metastases created a medical emergency necessitating Danny's return to the hospital. When I saw him next he was deeply depressed.

"I did everything the way I was supposed to. And then this happened. It is not fair."

"Cancer does not play fair," I replied. Danny asked what he could do.

"How about trying a 'so what' attitude. Maybe you will live until next year, maybe you won't. But in the meantime, live every minute fully. Be like a sponge and absorb the essence of every minute you have. If it makes you sad to think about not being here next year, don't think about it."

Danny agreed to wear a loose rubber band around his wrist. Whenever he caught himself thinking thoughts that made him sad, he snapped the rubber band against his wrist.

"Plan for the future if you must," I suggested, "but make your future one minute from now. The longest plan can be about this evening — who will come up to visit you. Make this day count. If

you want a certain person to come up to the hospital, call and make your wishes known. And then when your friend arrives, try to enjoy every single second. Look at the minute details of the face, the gestures made while talking."

Then Danny asked, *"But how do I make moments count when I am alone?"*

"You could look out of the window and record every detail of what you see. The tall buildings of downtown form the background. They are billowing smoke up into the sky like artillery. Take a look at those clouds and how they change form. And how about those older houses and apartment buildings on the fringe of the University campus?"

Danny got involved with our task, *"I remember some of those houses from when I was a young boy. Did you know I grew up not far from here?"* Danny then talked of his childhood and some of the adventures he had in this neighborhood. He was looking back into his life for the good times, the meaningful times.

Cancer patients take stock of their life. They accept life's good moments and bad. They accept it all, including the cancer.

Danny had resolved most of his conflicts very soon after our talk. Once he began using some of the power he still had to make his environment the way he wanted it, the depression lifted. Danny moved through the stages much faster than most people do, though he spent a lot of time in denial. Maybe when he moved, he was truely ready to grow. Yet Danny's family played an active role in helping him see a change was needed. He died a tranquil man. Had he remained in denial, I think he would have panicked toward the end. This way, he had time to get his emotions and his life in order.

Hostility

Hostility is the reaction that followed repression in most of my patients. Too many things start to go wrong, and the denial attitude cannot be maintained in the face of so much evidence to the contrary. The patient is overwhelmed by the unfairness of death and lashes out at any available target. The nurses are clumsy, the doctors incompetent. At home the food tastes rotten, the

daughter's new boyfriend is a fool. The patient does not want to
be reminded to take pills but he gets angry if the pills are forgotten. He wants his condition not to be fussed over, but heaven
forbid he should be ignored.

Hostility is hard for those around the patient to handle. It
seems unjust to the family. It is hard not to take the anger personally, even if you know it is coming from the cancer and not
from anything you did.

Several coping strategies are helpful for the second phase. One
is to work at not taking the anger personally. When you feel angry,
say to yourself, "I can handle this calmly. The cancer is the real
problem." Another strategy is to see things from the patient's
perspective. Repeat aloud what you think the patient is feeling.
"You feel we do not care for you because we talk to each other
outside your room and you feel left out." Finally, since hostility
is hard on the patient and the family, all should be done to move
through this stage as quickly as possible. This is accomplished
by dealing directly with the root of the hostility — the unfairness
of having to die.

In the hostility phase, the patient is feeling unjustly treated.
The patient complains that the doctor, nurses, and family members are treating him unjustly, but subconsciously he feels unjustly
treated by Fate or the cancer.

*My father was furious that he went through the ordeal of
chemotherapy for nothing. When he finished his treatments, he
came upon a magazine article that said chemotherapy is seldom
successful for intestinal cancer. He felt duped into being a guinea
pig when it could not help him. No one had an answer for his
complaint.*

Sometimes the family gets wrapped up in the patient's anger.
One mother was convinced the chemotherapy had weakened her
son and injured his liver to the extent that it was the chemotherapy that was killing him, not the cancer. She treated the
doctors who were trying to help as though they were murderers.

There are elements of helplessness and projection in the hostility. A bedridden patient is able to do very little for himself. Yet
the patient feels everyone else is incompetent. The steady loss
in the ability to do things someone has done all his life leads to a

great deal of frustration and irritability.

The family must try hard not to take the hostility personally. The patient is fighting against the realization that he or she will soon have to leave everything treasured. No matter what the patient does, the end is approaching with increasing urgency. All of a sudden life becomes very precious.

One way of moving the patient through this hostility as quickly as possible is to provide an outlet for the anger. Just be there and listen. At first allow the anger to come out. It is kind of like lancing a wound when you let the poisons seep out unhindered. With highly verbal patients, the angry outbursts can be vicious. You have to remember that anger is not nice. With quietly angry patients who seldom give themselves the right to hostility you have to help them voice their anger. You say what you think the patient is thinking because he cannot say it himself. But avoid preaching.

Anna was an elderly patient in a terminal ward of a hospital. When I first saw her, she was livid, but her lips were pressed together tight and she would not say a thing. Before going through the formalities of who I was and what I was doing there, I just said, "Something has really irritated you!" She started to deny it, but then she plainly agreed. "Yes, the nurses here just do not know how to provide care," she said.

I used a technique called active listening where you paraphrase what the person just said. You do this to let the patient come up with his own reasons and answers, since you do not have them.

"The nurses don't pay any attention to you," I said.

"That is right," Anna said, glad I did not try to talk her out of her belief. At first when working with an angry person, let them ventilate their feelings. Let them think what they want to think. Do not try to convince them of your beliefs.

Anna was not going to make it easy for me by telling me exactly what she meant by improper care. So I asked "What else do they do?"

"You tell me," she said combatantly with her brown eyes flashing from under her disarrayed white hair.

"It does not look like they come to the room very often."

"You can say that again. A person could just die here and no one would notice."

Dying patients have a strong fear of abandonment. When a terminally ill patient is complaining about the nurses, you can be pretty sure that their own family is not around. The real fear is isolation.

I asked Anna if there was any way I could help. She said there was nothing I could do. This is typical of angry patients who want your help but cannot ask for it and cannot accept help when it is given. You must persist.

"How about if I call your family and tell them you want a visit?"

She shook her head vigorously. "No, they are all too busy. Everyone works, you know. Nobody has time for me."

When she commented that no one had time for her, Anna's feelings about what angered her were apparent. Nurses were forgotten.

"I do not know your family, Anna, but is it possible they stay away because they just do not know how to handle your illness? Maybe they stay away because they care so much it gives them pain to come. Or maybe they just do not know what you want."

Anna thought this over, her lips still tightly clamped together. At her request, I talked to the family. They had been avoiding her at the hospital because Anna told them to stay away. "I need my rest," Anna insisted, thinking she was providing them with the out they wanted. When the family replied that she was no bother, Anna said they kept her awake when she wanted to sleep. She admitted to me that she did not need rest. She just did not want to be a burden on her family.

Anna wanted to see her family. They wanted to see her. But instead of making their desires known, they gave each other mixed messages.

Family communication breakdowns are common. People say what they think others want to hear rather than the message they wish to convey. Hostile or depressed patients frequently isolate themselves or banish certain members of the family. They test the limits of what others can take. The family must continue to provide support for the patient by just being around.

After we worked out the mixed message Anna had sent, her family timed their visits so Anna was never alone nor was she overwhelmed by too many visitors. Sometimes the visitors just sat by her bedside reading or doing homework while holding her hand. Her sister constantly fussed over Anna, braiding her hair, straightening her room. The two young grandchildren played with plastic toy soldiers on her bed with Anna's legs under the blanket positioned as mountains.

Hostile patients often cannot say what really troubles them. Instead they pick at inconsequential aspects of their existence: food is tasteless, TV is boring, the staff are incompetent. One way to help anger dissipate is to put in words what the patient is angry about. With cancer patients, it is easy to guess what is causing the irritability. Say something like

"You are angry you are ill."

"You wish things didn't turn out like this."

"There are things you still want to do."

It is best to make statements, not ask questions. The first time you make a statement illustrating you understand the patient's anger, the patient is apt either to look up at you with surprise or to let loose with a stream of pent up anger. When the anger comes, hold the patient's hand and quietly listen. Do not try to talk the patient out of his anger. I think anyone who is dying with cancer has a right to feel cheated. Let the patient have his feelings.

Some family members handle their hurt, which is what anger comes from, by thinking things such as "We all have to go sometime," "He is going to a better place," or "It is God's will." While these statements may bring you solace, the patient must find his or her own solacing statements. Generally, it is better to sit quietly, to listen, and to make statements like

"It's a shame,"

"What a horrible thing to happen," or

"It does seem unfair."

As the patient works through the anger, he will generate his own strategies for dealing with the tragedy. When he finds his solace, he will say something similar to

"Well, I guess everybody's got to die eventually." Then you can rub the patient's arm and say

"That's true." Letting the patient find his own answer, unless he asks you for yours, is the best strategy.

Hostility is a process. The patient is angry because he realizes his own death is likely. Before a patient can accept death, he has to admit the likelihood of death. This is why hostility presents progress toward acceptance. Even though repression is a more pleasant stage, which is easier on the patient and the family, hostility is progress because the patient is starting to realize that he is going to die. He does not like it, but he knows it is going to happen. Next, it is likely that this realization will depress him, but finally, he will accept it and the anguish will diminish. Even though an element of hope will persist, the patient will live for the moment rather than for something scheduled to occur two years hence. He will accept his life such as it is; he will accept the past with its good and bad moments, and he will accept whatever the future holds.

Sally was a twenty-nine-year-old nurse with leukemia. When the diagnosis was first confirmed, she was frantic looking for a way out. From her medical experience, she knew she faced an uphill battle with a lot to go through in terms of coping with the rigors of chemotherapy. She doubted whether she was strong enough emotionally to accept losing her hair, vomiting, and other reactions she had seen other patients have. She pondered returning to her former husband. At long last after many tears, Sally realized that she had the strength to face it alone.

"I still have hope," she said with conviction. "It is more than that — I firmly believe there is a cure for my kind of leukemia just around the corner. And I intend to stay alive until that cure is found."

Sally has changed her life around. She rigorously follows the diet her doctor prescribed and takes her chemotherapy without fail.

"This is a funny time in my life," she relates. "I have moments of the deepest despair, yet I have never been happier. I do only what I really want to do. If I want to call a friend long distance, I do it. I don't wait for the rates to change. I am trying to squeeze in everything I want to do because I know there are no guarantees for me."

Searching

The searching phase develops as a way to handle hostility. Instead of living with the impending possibility of death, the patient tries to eliminate death permanently or hold it in abeyance. Sometimes rather than magically eliminating the cancer, the patient will try to bargain away the pain, at least for a little while. Sometimes the patient succeeds in putting off death until some task is finished.

Searching patients seek out a magic cure. It may be laetrile, an anticancer diet, or a certain mineral water with curative powers. Patients eagerly read newspaper accounts of people who beat cancer by following some regimen. The patient tries it, denies bad symptoms, and clings to good days as evidence that the regimen is working. Desperate searching of this type is similar to denial except that now the patient acknowledges that the cancer does exist.

Other patients bargain for a little more time to finish an important task. They try to keep themselves in shape to keep up strength for a particular event.

Myrna's youngest daughter was quite broken up by her mother's illness. When Myrna was nursed at her other daughter's home, the youngest daughter was too distraught to help. She cried and cried through every visit. She was pregnant and the family feared Myrna's death might cause the daughter to loose the baby. Myrna was expected to die within the month and the baby was not due for three months. I was present the night Myrna told her weeping daughter that she would be around to see the baby.

The next day Myrna started exercising and sitting in the sun to keep her strength up. When the baby was born prematurely two months later, Myrna was there to admire the newborn. Myrna told me, "Now I can leave. My daughter has someone to love now. I promised I would go quietly if I could just please have the time until the baby came. I could have made it another month if I had to, you know." I believed her.

Like shock, searching is basically a somewhat happy phase, happier than hostility or despair. Bargaining is a time of hope, hope that some formula for prolonging life exists. Sometimes bargaining takes place when the patient still feels well. It is easy to think the bargain is working successfully under those circumstances.

Psychological intervention is not indicated when a patient is in the searching phase. It is not an unpleasant time for the patient or the family. Bargaining days are usually good days because the patient is seeking solutions and investigating alternative blueprints for living. The patient must consider every option and rule out all blind alleys. Some patients come to the realizations that dying is just another phase of living and that the answer is to get everything out of the remaining time. These patients go directly from searching to adjustment. Most patients, however, do not. Instead, the usual course is for a patient to perceive his bargains as futile. This makes the patient sad, and he slips into a state of hopelessness and despair.

Despair

The patient who is sad is grieving for himself and all he is soon to loose. There are many legitimate reasons for being depressed. When you think about how sad you are that you are going to lose the one you love, consider how very much more sad the patient must be that he or she is going to lose you, everyone else, every experience ever known and the option for further experiences. Also, the patient fears what he or she may have to go through in the final states of the terminal illness. "How much pain can I tolerate?" the patient asks. The patient knows he or she will be totally dependent on others for care, and he cannot be sure he will not be abandoned to the care of strangers when the going gets rough.

One depressed patient told me that everything in life suddenly became more precious to her when she discovered she had terminal cancer. Every breeze from the window, every look around the room was worth more to her than all the money in the world. She had always loved sunsets and rainbows but now she had no guarantee that she would live to see another. It seemed that her sense of smell and hearing were more acute, and she reveled in sensory experiences as she had never done before.

She was clinging to life, clutching to every experience precious to her. I think for her and many depressed patients the answer to their despair is letting go. The cancer patient must accept death, they must let go of the things and people they love. The sunset may be appreciated with joy whether it is the last sunset to be seen or not. Good-byes are said to places much as one does when moving away from a town.

Again, the patient's challenge is to work through the despair, coming to his own resolution. The sadness must be expressed, not repressed. If the patient is told "Don't feel bad," he or she is apt to put the despair down far inside himself and be caught in this phase for a long time, perhaps the rest of his life.

Verbal explanations appeal to the intellectual part of us. Despair stems from our emotional being. If we are going to help, we must appeal to the emotional part on the person. One of the best ways is to be present and just hold hands with the patient. Stroke the patient's arm or caress his head with a wet cloth. Verbal explanations will not help. Physical contact which conveys emotional support and caring works better.

Sometimes contact with other terminal patients can help. There are groups with names such as "I Can Cope" and "Make Today Count" with chapters in cities across the nation. The latter group was started by a terminal cancer patient named Orville Kelly and his wife Wanda. Orville, a man in his forties with terminal cancer, little financial security, and four growing children, found the key to his depression was getting the most out of the remaining time and not mourning for what he could not have. Don't think coming to this resolution was quick for him. Group support from people who understand and are coping with the problem may help. A good place to start is checking out Kelly's book from the public library.

If the patient remains in despair for a long time, say a month, or does not have much time left to work it out, I think it makes sense to help the patient work through the sadness and make progress toward resolving the conflict.

You can begin by making statements expressing what you see happening. These statements should be nonjudgemental and very sympathetic. You accept what the patient is feeling and give your permission for having those feelings. The patient has every right to those feelings and, in point of fact, does not need your permission to have them, but often the patient feels better knowing these negative feelings are perfectly normal and understandable. You convey your understanding when you say

"You are very sad."

"The thought of leaving us makes you sad."

"Everything seems hopeless to you."

Sometimes the depressed patient will open up after one of these statements and share his feelings. Other times, the patient may just cry. Either response is beneficial for the patient because feelings are getting out. When someone cries, you may hold the person close and cry along with him.

Another way to help the patient work through the despair is to share your feelings in terms of I-messages:

"I get so sad when I think I may not have you with me forever."

"I know I'll always have you with me in my heart, but sometimes I get selfish and want more."

"I wish I could go through this for you. At least I can promise that I will go through this with you."

"I treasure every moment with you."

Then sit next to the patient, hold his or her hand, and wait. Cry if you feel like it; it is very therapeutic at this point. Just do not run away. The patient may not be able to respond at first, but eventually he will in words or tears. Then you will know you have made contact, breaking through the wall of hopelessness, the root of this phase.

Despair is hard for relatives to cope with. Family members feel very sorry for the cancer patient and also for themselves. Any sign someone is unhappy makes us uncomfortable and sometimes makes us want to leave and not see the pain. The important thing about despair is not to take it personally. Accept the depression as a genuine, predictable feeling. Help get the emotions expressed. Help also by remaining with the patient. Depressed patients sometimes do not converse much. Do not feel you have to fill the void with words. Just being there is enough.

If the patient cannot express feelings, you can try doing it for him. My father was silently depressed for a long time so I tried to express what I thought were his feelings.

"Are you feeling sad, Dad?"

"Yes, a little."

"I was thinking how depressing it is for me to think about someday maybe being parted from you. But it must be much harder and sadder for you to think about having to leave all of us."

During this time my sister Bonnie noticed how aware Dad seemed to be of us. He would maintain eye contact when talking, but could not talk long because tears came to his eyes. He thoroughly enjoyed his grandchildren, but only for a little while. Then he retreated to his bedroom. I think we were much more precious to him than ever before, but he was also much saddened by the thought of leaving us.

Another time I asked, *"Are you afraid, Dad?"* He replied that he was not, which is the socially acceptable answer to this question, but his facial expression said something else. Later I defined my questions more closely and asked, *"Are you afraid of the pain, Dad?"*

This time he replied affirmatively. *"Yes, I am. I read in a magazine that it gets real bad in cancer patients. Last night it was bad."*

"Night is a frightening time. We will do everything we can to help you like staying with you all night. One person will always be next to your bed. There are some ways of lessening pain that we will try. Can you let us know when you are in pain?"

"Yes, I could ring my bell if you're not here."

"That's a good idea, but we will be here. Also, I will talk to the doctor about your medication and see if he thinks it should be changed. Is there anything else I can do to help?"

"Don't leave me alone. I am afraid you will all leave when it gets bad."

"You will never be alone. I promise you that. Do you think about what it is like to die?"

"Yes, I wonder what it is like."

"I read some reports by people who experienced clinical death and later were resuscitated. These people all agreed that dying was a pleasant experience. It looks as if the brain plays out all the beautiful memories of a lifetime just before the end."

"That doesn't sound so bad."

"No, I did not think so," I replied.

"I think I could face it that way," my father said.

At the end of the phase of despair, Dad was talking about meeting us later on the other side of a particular fence he had to climb. The symbolism, of course, was about dying. He had found a way to come to grips with leaving us.

The end of this phase of hopelessness marks the ability of the patient to dissociate himself from his body. Emotionally, the patient no longer clings to his physical form but is able to part from it and get away from pain and sickness. The patient says good-bye to places and accepts the fact that he has to face parting from loved ones. Hope comes in feeling that memories will live on.

In my work I have met patients who do not have religious feelings about life after death. These patients also resolve their despair by accepting the release that death will bring. They do not speak about meeting with family members after death. Instead, they concentrate on memories of the good times they had in life and find solace in what they did and what will remain after they are gone.

Adjustment

The goal in the process of coming to grips with dying is the adjustment to the inevitable. The patient realizes he can part with his family, and he has emotionally parted from his body. There is a feeling that there is more to a person than just a body, which serves as a shell. The present body has outlived its usefulness.

Patients who have resolved conflicts about dying are in a neutral peace, devoid of strong feelings. The patient loves his family but does not cling to them as before. The stage of adjustment characteristically is more than resignation. It is not a sad phase, nor is it happy. Strong emotional turmoil is over; business is finished.

In my family, we all achieved adjustment about the same time. This was nice because we could deal with aspects of dying without anyone falling apart. Sometimes all of us still had periods of tears;

this is normal, but what we felt was not the heart-rendering an-
guish we felt in the previous stages. You see, we too had accepted
Dad's death and were willing to let him go with love.

One day Dad interrupted me while I was reading aloud a
newspaper to him.

"Let's not waste time."

"OK, Dad. What do you want to talk about?"

"I know I am going to die."

"I know it too. How can I help?"

"When the time comes, let me go."

"I will. We all have accepted the way things are and will stay
with you. When the time comes for you to go, we will let you go
with love."

"Even your mother?"

"Even Mother. We spoke about it last night."

"Good, I needed to know that."

After this conversation, Dad no longer had trouble with pain.
I do not know why. Perhaps the tension of fighting death made
him uncomfortable. He seemed to be released from his body and
his suffering. He stopped talking much and used gestures for
communicating. He smiled when we conversed with him. He held
hands with us and kissed us when we helped him. When I told him
I would have him forever in my heart, he smiled and patted his
chest nodding affirmatively.

Once Dad accepted dying, it seemed that the rest of us fol-
lowed along with the tension of death being over. We all had the
inner conviction that our memories of him and our inner relation-
ship with him would live on. Those last days were easier for him
and for us than the trying days of depression or anger. Now we
were just biding time, keeping Dad comfortable and using those
final precious moments remaining to show him our love.

In the stage of adjustment everything falls into place and
makes sense. Each family member's conception of life and death
is different since it depends on background and philosophical
beliefs. It is necessary to realize that dying is just the final stage of
living. Dying is not separate from living but rather is another part
of living with its own special joys and sorrows. Death is nothing
more than part of the continuous process of life. This final time in

life may be successful as previous stages were.

My father died with a great deal of dignity. He lived fully up to the final moment. He continued to treat us with respect as we did him. His death was peaceful and beautiful. In dying he taught me a great deal about courage that I intend to use in my own time.

Who Will Not Reach Adjustment

For some patients there is not adequate time to work through all the stages before the death. Accident patients or those with a fast-moving tumor may die in the shock of denial. These patients are spared the rigors of the phases of hostility and despair.

Even with intensive counseling, not every patient or family member will reach the stage of adjustment. Some people die angry or depressed. There are several reasons why this happens.

For some people anger is their characteristic way of handling not only a crisis but also everyday living. It is likely these people will not reach adjustment. Anger is too much a part of them to feel something else so late in the game. The same holds true of people who are chronically depressed. Sometimes this boomerangs.

One of my patients, Martha, was single and middle-aged when I first saw her. Her family was exasperated with her. Martha could best be described as sniveling. She complained constantly and manipulated her family with her depressions. Whenever they did not do what she wanted, Martha tried suicide or something else equally hysterical. Martha was a difficult patient to work with, and I must confess I was not successful with her. Martha refused all therapy, preferring instead her passive-aggressive ways of making people do what she wanted. When she had to be hospitalized, Martha's depression subsided. She had been right: someday her family would be sorry for all the wrongs they committed against her. At first, Martha was happy in the hospital with nurses at her beck and call; later she felt they were avoiding her. Martha never reached the adjustment stage. Her depression returned and remained with her for the rest of her days.

How Much to Tell the Patient

There is quite a bit of controversy regarding how much to tell the cancer patient about his illness. Do you tell him he has cancer? Do you tell him it is malignant and has spread? What if he wants to know how much time is left?

In the past, patients were told as little as possible. This secrecy stemmed from diverse reasons. It was thought to be more humane not to tell the whole truth. The goal was to give patients hope and keep them from becoming depressed. In fact, this approach was the easy way out for family members and doctors because it is much simpler to say something good, even if it is not true, than to say something bad. Another reason for the subterfuge was that doctors really did not know how much time was left or what the progress of the disease would be.

Some patients want the truth; others do not want to know. I believe that you do what the patient wants. If the patient does not want to know anything, say nothing. Do not lie, just say nothing. It is cruel to push bad news on someone who cannot cope with it. If the patients wants the truth, tell him the whole truth as you know it. Never lie or the patient will find it hard to believe what you say.

Patients have ways of discovering the truth. A chart is read when it is accidently left in the examining room with the patient or sent with the patient down to X-ray. A patient reads a letter from a relative who talks about the cancer thinking the patient has been informed. Even young children with leukemia find out what disease they have. On their own they proceed to read up about the disease. Parents who mistakenly think the child is uninformed are flabbergasted at the extent of information the child has accumulated. Even a child can figure out that something pretty serious must be wrong to warrant all the hospital stays, treatments, and hair falling out. They cannot be expected to go through the ordeal without some explanation.

I have never known a patient who was lied to who did not guess the truth. After figuring out the truth, the patient invariably reacts with anger and depression. The patient's anger and depression are augmented by being lied to. The bond of basic trust between the patient and his family is damaged, sometimes broken.

At this point patients angrily denounce the fact that they were not told. "I could have used my time so much better. Now I have wasted all these months," is a typical response. Patients want to be part of the decision-making process. After all, he or she is the one who is going through the discomfort of the tests, radiation, or chemotherapy. It is only fair that the patient should know what he or she is getting into and how it is apt to turn out. Otherwise, the patient will feel cheated and betrayed.

When I am involved in telling a patient something, I first ask them how much they want to know. Quite often the patient asks me to hold off until they get psychologically prepared. I think this is fair, so I wait until the patient is ready.

Of course, when a patient is told that he has metastatic cancer, depression or hostility may follow after an initial period of shock and denial. There is no way around the hopelessness and hostility, and anger, no matter how the news is broken or covered up. Do not be afraid of anger or sadness, or feel guilty when the patient has negative feelings. Anyone with cancer has every right in the world to feel angry or sad. This is part of the process that leads to adjustment and the desire to make the most of the time remaining.

I know it is not easy to tell a loved one about a metastatic cancer diagnosis. But believe me, it is much harder to live a lie. You have to watch everything you say or do every single minute of the day. You must be on your guard to warn everyone the patient talks to not to say anything. You must vigilantly monitor incoming and outgoing mail and keep posted over the telephone so the extension is not picked up at the wrong time. This kind of vigilance uses up too much of your energy in a nonproductive manner.

We are increasingly less willing to tolerate not being told the truth. Perhaps we are going back to the pioneer values of truthfulness and honesty. They are not such bad values. Things are much easier when you only have to remember one version.

Remember, by adjusting, the patient does not lose hope. Reasonable medical procedures are tried. But if the procedures do not work, the other alternative can be accepted, also. In the meantime, life will be lived and enjoyed even in a limited capacity.

When you consider what chemotherapy takes out of a person or the side effects of radiation, I do not see how you can expect a person to go through it without understanding the situation. How could you resolve the inconsistency of telling a patient that there was nothing wrong with her but she had to take this medicine that would make her vomit for six months?

A person has a right to decide under what circumstances life is worth living. Sometimes people are not willing to suffer for six months so that they can live under diminised capacity for two months. Growth of brain tumors, for instance, is slowed after chemotherapy so the patient can live longer. But sometimes by the time the growth is retarded, much damage has been done. The patient may not be able to walk, speech may be slurred, or the functioning in the arm or the whole half of the body may be drastically impaired. I believe the patient has a right to choose whether he wants to go on that way. Maybe chemotherapy to prolong this kind of life is not worth it. Nobody can make that decision but the patient.

In my experience, a fair share of patients with metastatic cancer will choose not to hear anymore news about the progress of terminal illness after they are told the cancer has spread, and I firmly believe that you respect the patient's rights to hear no more bad news. The patient knows the bottom line; why remind him of it?

An oncologist told me an interesting story about an eighty-year-old man who had cancer of the colon, much advanced. The family told the doctor not to tell the old man because he might not be able to take it. The doctor believed his ethics required him to speak directly to his patient and not to the family until he had the patient's permission. The old man took the news well, saying he had lived a long and full life. He refused further treatment. "I won't last a year, will I, Doctor?" the man asked. The doctor thought more like a half a year given the state of the cancer. "I knew it before the exam. And don't tell my family, I want them to be happy and treat me like they always did," was the patient's last statement. The old man died peacefully. The moral of his story is that you cannot always tell how someone will respond to bad news.

Chapter 5

MAINTAINING INTEGRITY

A S time passes, terminal patients face a growing sense of inability to control their environment. Their impact on the world around them and their control of what is happening to their body diminish. The sense of independence in making free choices is continually eroded. Patients become increasingly less mobile and may even regress to the distressing point of not being able to manage bodily functions.

Although most terminal cancer patients end up bedridden, their mental capacities are usually unimpaired. People caring for a terminal patient should help the patient to retain a feeling of control. Some ways this can be accomplished include maintaining the predictability of the environment, the ability to make choices, the opportunity for movement, and continued attention to appearance.

Another area where the patient must maintain some control is the area of knowing what will happen to his or her body. The patient is apprehensive of what his internment will be like and how death will feel. These are hard questions to answer because no one knows for sure.

People who provide the care are mainly responsible for helping the patient to maintain a feeling of integrity. Feelings of integrity come from within, but they are also a reflection of how the patient perceives the outside world acting toward him.

The person who provides care has more contacts with the patient in the course of daily living than anyone else and can actively work to let the patient make as many choices as possible about food, clothing, visitors, and just day-to-day living. The environment should be predictable with a daily routine followed in the same way one was followed before the patient got sick. The patient should be treated as though he still matters. At the very least, friends and relatives can serve as sounding boards so the patient can verbalize his fears.

Predictability

Knowing what will happen and when provides comfort. Security results from operating with certainty in the environment and taking comfort in its predictability. A schedule followed closely day after day helps the patient know when to expect things, just as a schedule during healthy years helped the patient get to work or school on time and organize his life. A daily schedule also reduces a patient's dependence. The patient will not demand a bath at a potentially inconvenient time if he knows that a bath always follows breakfast. Setting up a communication system that works predictably relieves tension.

Whenever Dad wanted company he rang a bell on the wall by his bed. The reasons he rang it varied. Sometimes he was in pain, sometimes he wanted a drink or needed to be moved, and other times he just felt a little lonely or frightened and needed company. The fact that someone always came immediately when he rang the bell made him secure knowing he was not abandoned even when no one was in sight. At night the bell woke us even when we were sleeping in another part of the house. We slept soundly in the knowledge that we could be in our own beds and still hear him when he rang.

Robert lived through the terminal phase of his bout with cancer exhibiting the same pattern of self-sufficiency he had shown all his life in other endeavors. Overall, he did not have continuous pain, just occasional spasms. When he got spasms, he needed support and help from his family, but he could not ask for it. Instead his teeth could clamp together and his body would tense up, making the pain all the worse. I gave Robert a special pain bell to alert his family. Since he used it only when he was in pain that he could not manage, the family always came running to see if they could help. They knew Robert would not speak, so they decided between themselves on their strategy for helping him handle it. Sometimes they gave him an injection; other times they continued with diversionary tactics until the spasm passed. Robert appreciated their attention and not having to talk to get it. He felt secure in his environment because he knew that he would get assistance when needed.

Daily Routine

Although daily routines will vary from patient to patient, typically the day will start with the relative or a nurse bringing the patient the necessary implements to wash himself, clean his teeth and comb his hair. Let the patient do as much for himself for as long as possible. Do not bother to change pajamas or bedding at this point. Give breakfast first. Sit down while the patient is eating, have coffee yourself, and read the morning paper aloud. Some patients enjoy watching the news or a morning television show during breakfast.

After breakfast, the morning sponge bath can be completed and fresh pajamas donned. Now is a good time to change the linen, since it may be damp. This can be done with the bedridden patient rolled to the far side of the bed while the caretaker completely re-sheets half of the bed. The patient is then rolled to the clean side while the caretaker completes the job on the other side.

After a night's sleep, breakfast, and bath, the patient is refreshed and ready to do something. Midmorning is a good time for visitors, a ride outside in the wheelchair, or a snooze in the sun. Pain is generally least in the morning, and energy is at its highest point. A patient who knows for sure that he will get out each day looks forward to this time. Most people find mornings better for doctors appointments than afternoons when the patient is more tired.

Throughout the day give the pain medication only on demand unless the patient is taking a medication such as morphine for continuous pain, which necessitates strict adherence to a schedule. If the patient is scheduled for a trip to the doctor, plan to give a shot about twenty minutes before you leave. The patient should then be able to tolerate the jostling of the trip and whatever examination procedures the doctor uses. If visitors are expected to come, try to arrange the shot schedule so the patient will not be in pain during the visit. You might have to give a shot a little bit early to insure comfort so the patient can enjoy the visit. If the patient always falls asleep after a shot, the dosage may be too great. See if your doctor approves giving less medication or breaking the large dose down into more frequently given smaller amounts.

Try to serve lunch with the patient sitting in the wheelchair. It makes for a nice change after having breakfast in bed. Changing positions is excellent for the patient's circulation and also tires him a bit so he is more prone to an afternoon nap. While the patient sleeps, the caretaker should also rest, especially if you have to get up at night to help the patient.

Breaking up the long afternoon is a matter of many small activities. Getting the patient up after the nap, rinsing his mouth out with mouthwash and combing the hair put a definite finish to the nap, avoiding the bad habit of cat napping all day and then not being able to sleep at night. Next the patient could listen to his or her favorite music for awhile. An afternoon tea where the caretaker sits down and reads the day's mail or newspaper provides structure to this time block.

Afternoon is a good time for friends to help out. If the friends do not know what to say, they can read to the patient or just sit and listen to the music. During the evening, friends who work can visit, but the patient will often be exhausted by then and testy from dealing with pain all day.

For friends who do not know what to do or say for a patient who really does not want visitors, you are in kind of a bind. Of course, your first loyalties and responsibilities are with the patient. But you might try putting the friend to work on some repair project or errand that needs attention. The "Friends" section gives some suggestions as to what these projects could be. Doing this keeps the friend busy and happy, gives the patient his privacy as well as the security knowing the friend is around and still cares.

The evening meal can be followed by the evening news and perhaps more television or music. Some patients find an evening sponge bath relaxing.

The daily schedule will show some variation just due to our inability to completely control things. This will provide the necessary variety to avoid boredom. You find that the patient takes solace in knowing the structure of his day. Even if the routine tasks are mundane, the patient will look forward to them because they contribute to his sense of security.

Choices

As adults we all enjoy making independent choices. Cancer patients are loath to give up making choices about what they want to wear or eat, and it is healthier for them not to give up having preferences. Caretakers must work at giving the patient the opportunity to make as many choices as possible for as long as possible. After the morning bath, let the patient choose which pajama top or shirt to wear.

An old doctor friend who had worn a tie everyday of his life for the past fifty years continued to wear a tie while bedridden with prostate cancer. He appreciated receiving gifts of after shave lotion and stationery. "I still matter," was all he said.

There are many things to make a choice about: what television programs to watch, which people to invite over to visit, what time to tell the visitors to come, how to plan tomorrow's routine, what roads to take to the doctor's office, and more.

Although Dad was on a liquid diet, we let him plan his diet around the foods he could have. We tried to keep many different kinds of fruit juices and soda pop on hand so he could try a new kind each day. We accented all the positive choices he could make rather than all the things he could not have.

It takes more time to ask the patient what his or her choices are than it would take to make the choice yourself. But by letting the patient choose, sometimes forcing them to choose, "Who do you want over tonight? Jim or Betty?", you are showing the patient that he still matters. You should also be willing to go along with his decision to see no one. His opinion still counts. What he thinks is important. He is not dead yet.

Helping the Patient Move Around

Helping the patient move is another way of showing him that he still matters. Letting the patient lay in the bed all day without moving diminishes his sense of living. You can imagine how depressed you would become if you were not allowed out of bed again, ever.

Putting a daily walk on your schedule helps. The patient knows that no matter what, he will get outside each day. At first, the patient may protest at letting others see him or her in a wheelchair. But soon the advantages of getting out in the sun, hearing the birds, seeing the landscape will outweigh any disadvantages. The patient will appreciate each little piece of beauty around him. You and the patient will have new things to talk about. When the patient's condition deteriorates, he may say good-bye to a certain garden, view, or walk and refuse to go back again. Respect the patient's wishes in this case and stop the walk.

Most daily routines are helped by the patient knowing that at certain times he will be in a different locale. The patient can be moved to a different room or put in front of the television for awhile. Before lunch perhaps the patient would enjoy sitting with you in the kitchen watching you prepare food.

Let the patient choose to lie down flat or be in a sitting position. As time goes on and he spends more and more of his day in bed, positioning becomes more important. Positioning includes rolling the patient from one side to the other or pulling him up to a sitting or standing position. Changing positions promotes circulation and takes the pressure off cramped organs.

Having a hospital bed with a head and feet portion that can be lowered or raised helps tremendously. However, you can manage without a hospital bed by pulling the patient to a new position and propping him up with pillows. The patient can help pull himself up by the use of a rope or sheet tied to the foot of the bed.

Turning the patient to his side provides pleasant relief to the overused skin on the back. Turn the patient on his side, place a pillow between his legs, another by his chest to prevent him from turning too far and a third behind his back so he will not unexpectedly roll backwards. While you have him on his side, massage the skin on the back. Those areas which are reddened and wrinkled need extra lotion and massaging, although you must show care in not breaking this skin by rubbing too hard.

Lying prone on the stomach is another possibility, but one not recommended for patients with abdominal or colon cancers and distended stomachs. If you try this position, put a pillow under the abdomen or chest for greater comfort. Watch for difficulties with breathing in this position.

Dad had some trouble breathing a couple of times when he was sitting upright. Apparently, when he was sitting, his abdomen would fill with fluids, which pushed against his lungs, cramping them. Carol, the R.N. who taught us so much about nursing, laid him back down flat with only one pillow and spoke reassuringly to him until his panic about being short of breath subsided. This illustrates the importance of changing positions frequently.

To make movement easier, try to tie a heavy knotted rope to the foot of the bed. The patient can grasp it to pull himself into a sitting position. A knotted bed sheet would serve the same function. A trapeze secured over the bed can also be used by the patient when pulling himself to a sitting position. How to secure the trapeze will be left up to your resourcefulness. Before you rent a hospital bed, see if you can get one with an overhead bar and trapeze attachment.

Moving the Patient

When you want to help a person move around, you must position yourself properly in order to get maximum leverage and also to protect your own muscles from strain. There are some general rules of body mechanics you may find helpful. Avoid back strain and injury by following these rules.

Stand close to your patient when you are moving him or her. Place your feet near his so you do not have to bend forward at the waist to get close. Position your feet under the bed, slightly turned toward the head of the bed. Rest your legs against the side of the bed to steady yourself.

Keep your back straight. You want to lift from the legs. You can do this only if you are standing close to the patient or close to the bed. When you go to lift, bend your legs from a deep knee bend position and stand straight up. If you bend over and pull upwards with your back, the back muscles will feel the strain. You keep your balance when lifting by keeping your feet apart with one foot ahead of the other. Tighten your muscles before use or exertion to avoid injuring them.

If you have to move something heavy, avoid lifting it. Instead try pulling it. Pulling is easier on your body than pushing, but both pushing and pulling are easier than lifting, which you should do only as a last resort. If you have to lift or carry something, keep it as close to your body as possible. Do not hold a heavy object far in front of you because it strains your muscles.

Whenever possible get assistance before moving the patient. I think one person can care for a patient by himself only as long as the patient can help himself a little. When it gets too much of a burden to move the patient, keep him in bed. Sponge baths, enemas, all functions can be provided for someone who cannot leave the bed. The main movement the patient will get when he is bedridden and has only one caretaker is being rolled from side to side or pulled to a sitting position. This movement is excellent and will suffice. If you really think the patient must get up or be transferred to a wheelchair, do it with a friend present to help. With two people, one under each of the patient's arms, the patient can be moved even when he cannot help himself much.

Before making a move, calmly tell the patient where you are going to move him and what you expect him to do to help. Even when the patient appears not to be lucid, he often still helps you to move him and follows your directions very well.

Use the weight of the patient to assist the movement. To move a patient up in the bed, have the patient lie on his back with his knees bent. Say, "I am going to move you farther up on the bed. When I count three, push yourself up toward the head of the bed. One, two, three, push!" You have your arms under his shoulders and the other under his things and you push upward on the count of three. If you have a cross sheet on the bed, you will find it invaluable in moving the patient up. The easiest way to move a patient up is to have two people, one on each side of the patient, pull up on a cross sheet on the count of three when the patient pushes with his feet. Also, be sure to tuck the cross sheet in securely to avoid wrinkles.

For any move, use your whole hand when you lift the patient. Avoid pulling him by the arms for fear of dislocating the shoulder. Also, watch that your fingers do not dig into the skin, causing bruising. Skin breaks do not heal easily.

Try to support the patient's joints and back during any movement. If the patient is moving himself, encourage him to push or pull, roll or slide. Hoisting himself up is potentially harmful.

After trying all methods just suggested, we found a cross sheet to be the best for pulling Dad up in bed or turning him to the side. One person stood at each side of the bed with feet properly placed. We counted to three, and pulled the cross sheet up while Dad pushed. He was supported in it like a babe in a hammock. Because our hands did not touch him during the move, we avoided all accidental scrapes such as rings scraping the skin and bruises from finger pressure.

Turning

To turn a patient, first remove all pillows and objects used for support. Cross one of the patient's legs over the other leg in the direction of the turn. Stand on the side of the bed the patient will face after the turn. Place your hands on the shoulder and hip on the side of the body away from you. Gently pull the body toward you. With very heavy patients, move the shoulder first and then the hip toward you, using both hands if necessary. After turning the shoulder, quickly prop it up with a pillow and then move the hip.

If you have an extra sheet crossways on the bed under the patient, you can use this to turn the patient. Stand on the side of the bed the patient will face after the turn. Reach across the patient and take the edges of the pull sheet. Pull it toward you until the patient is on his or her side.

You need not fear the patient will roll out of bed because you are standing at the edge. Prop the patient with pillows behind and in front so he or she cannot roll over the edge of the bed. If the bed has bedrails, always keep them up when the patient is on his side.

Friends

Close friends of the patient go through anticipatory grieving and turmoil just as the family members do. Friends need a chance to work through their grief and do something for the patient. While family members are together because of being related, the patient and his friends chose to be together because they liked each other's company. This puts friends in the rather unique situation of loving, caring but also feeling that they do not belong the way family members do.

My father had three close friends, Jack, Bob, and Ralph. Each man handled his grieving in a different way. Dad was able to interact with each man separately to help him at various stages of his quest for acceptance.

Jack and Dad were childhood friends in one of those friendships that persists quietly throughout the years. Jack was in my parent's wedding party and was also a pall bearer. The last time Jack and his wife saw Dad was during the late summer, six months before he died. Dad was vacillating between anger and depression and was probably not very good company. Jack went away, encapsulated his sorrow and had little further contact until the funeral where he cried and was obviously very sad. Jack did not go away because he did not care. He cared, but perhaps he did not know how to express it or how to help. Maybe he felt uncomfortable or unwanted. In any case, he chose to handle his feelings in private.

Another friend, Bob, who Dad knew almost as long as Jack, continued to visit Dad throughout his angry times. On the exterior Bob appears to be rather abrasively insensitive, but he is quite perceptive. Bob continued to visit Dad off and on, bringing him books and other things to occupy time even though Dad often asked him to leave. Bob never took Dad's bad moods personally and did not feel unwanted even when he was.

Ralph was a relatively new friend, having met Dad on the job in the last few years of his life. While working, Dad and Ralph had a lot of fun together and established the kind of warm and happy relationship one usually only gets while young. Ralph remained completely loyal to Dad throughout his internment. He tried to keep things going for Dad such as managing some unfinished business at work. Ralph and his wife Charlotte visited regularly, brought over food and coffee, and did any number of thoughtful tasks. Ralph was visibly suffering during my father's illness and even more so during the funeral. To this day Ralph is still helping the family in many important ways, as is Bob.

From these three different kinds of friends, one can see various reactions. The most typical is Jack. This is the friend who cares and is sad but does not know what to do about it. Old friends who have moved apart into separate life spaces are apt to fall into this category. I think there is nothing to do but let them go and work out their sorrow on their own.

Most friends will be like Bob, coming over from time to time. If you needed something done, he would do it, but on his own he probably will not think of the many little things you need. Friends like Bob are good sounding boards for the patient. They can take the anger or the depression and not be destroyed by it. In fact, they will come back for more.

If you have even one friend like Ralph, you are fortunate. Friends like Ralph sensitively anticipate your needs and give of themselves unselfishly. You can help with their anguish by giving them tasks. By doing and helping and working, they can find an outlet for their sorrow.

While none of Dad's friends were repelled by cancer, some people are. The effects can be startling, as one of my patient's discovered.

Everyone in her home town knew of Jill's cancer. At a Christmas party, Jill noticed that while all the other guests were drinking from glass cups, the hostess had given her a paper cup.

The whole topic of death is something some people will not deal with and do not want to see. These people you must definitely let go. There is not enough time left to waste it on someone whose development in this area is so egocentric and shallow.

Friends and relatives may call, ask how the patient is doing, and offer to help. There are good reasons for letting friends help when they offer. First, you may need some help — caring for a sick person is not easy — although you will be tempted to decline. Society trains us to be unrealistically self-reliant. Second, friends deserve to be given a chance to work through their grief. They cannot push themselves into the inner circle the way relatives can, they can only ask to help.

Our neighbors popped in with entire meals that tasted so good. One neighbor sent over a 3 pound can of coffee because she knew we were sitting up late with Dad. Charlotte and Ralph periodically sent cakes or other deserts. Seeing the gifts on the counter top was testimony to the silent support surrounding us. The friendship continued after Dad died. The mother of a childhood friend of mine babysat my young son the day of the funeral.

Do you need help? You think not, but let's face it: all the chores you and the sick person used to do around the house still need doing. And don't forget: you must take care of yourself during this demanding period. This means occasionally have fun, keep physically fit, read for pleasure, and get a haircut. Here are some suggestions of the type you can give to people who call offering help:

rake leaves
prune foliage
shovel snow off the sidewalk or driveway
wax the floors
take garbage out
make a small household repair
pick up a prescription
take the car in to get the oil changed
pick up clothes at the laundry
iron or wash clothes ·
bake a casserole or something nutritious
prepare a clear broth for the patient
wash and set your hair or the patient's hair
sit with the patient at night so you can sleep
do general housecleaning

Adapt this list to your own particular situation. The caretakers have tasks that need to be done that they will not get to. Friends want to help, so give them a chance. It is selfish to keep all the care in your own hands when others are feeling suffering and need a chance to work out their hurt.

What Friends Can Do if the Caretakers Turn Them Down

As a friend, you may call, offer assistance, and be turned down. What you can do is persist. Call back again, but do not ask the family what you can do — tell them what you are going to do.

"When I drove by this morning, I noticed the grass needs mowing. My son and I are coming over today to work on it. What time would be good so the mower won't disturb Frank?"

"I was putting together a casserole for dinner and put in an extra one for you. Is it convenient for me to drop it off now?"

"My kids and I are coming over to wash your windows. It's something we want to do for Ellen."

"I have made an appointment for you with the woman who does my hair. It is my treat. She understands the situation and will take you with no waiting. I will sit with Harry while you go."

There is so much that friends can do. Beyond their help, knowing the sincerity of their feelings provides warmth during the otherwise occasionally bleak times.

Chapter 6

WHAT DYING IS LIKE

THE act of dying is something unknown to most of us even though we have seen death portrayed in movies and have read about it in literature. Generations ago, dying was not so mysterious and frightening: death took place at home, life expectancy was shorter, and older relatives lived with younger families. We have chosen to insulate ourselves from death, thus perhaps making dying appear more gruesome than it needs to be.

What are you getting into by bringing a patient home to die? To relate what dying is like I spoke to many people who watched a loved one die. They all concurred that dying by cancer is not nearly as awesome as it is portrayed.

When you look at symptoms of dying, the most important variable is change. Sometimes, the process of change encompasses a complete loss of function. In the case of kidneys no longer functioning, death would be near. But more often it is change in the sense of functioning less well such as decreased output of urine from the kidneys. Or change could be new breathing patterns, such as Cheyne-Stoking, described later. So notice any change, particularly a change for the worse.

Urine

Excretion of waste is a vital bodily function. Urine excretion is more important for the body than bowel function. A person with total bowel blockage can live for some time with no bowel movement, providing no food is taken in, although this cannot go on indefinitely.

87

However, the body must output urine every day to survive. Urine excretion is the main way the body cleans itself of toxins and poisons. Renal failure is lethal.

When the kidneys start to fail, urine output will decrease. The total urine output for a day may drop to about a cupful. The urine will become very dark in color, most likely an orangey-red. It will also smell worse than ordinary urine. Another sign of weakening kidneys is swelling in the lower part of the groin.

Uremic poisoning is the name of the condition that exists when the kidneys begin to malfunction. Some of the symptoms include lassitude and fatigue. This quiet period presents a stark contrast to the previous complaining or burst of energy. The patient suddenly seems so much weaker and sleeps longer than he or she ever did before. Mental acuity is not as sharp as it used to be. The patient may not recognize some friends, although this may also be the result of being heavily medicated for a long time.

Other symptoms of uremic poisoning include muscles that twitch or cramp. This is caused by the increase of toxins in the body that the kidneys cannot excrete. The patient loses all desire for food and may vomit or become nauseated. Another sign of uremic poisoning is the skin turning yellow-brown. Sometimes the minerals not being secreted in the urine come through the skin and crystallize there. If this happens, wipe the skin off with a damp rag frequently to keep the patient from smelling.

As fluids build up, you will see swollen hands and feet and perhaps swelling in the abdomen. Excessive retention of sodium and water may lead to congestive heart failure. Sometimes a patient will convulse from the toxins in his system. Just quiet him and yourself. If this happens, make sure the breathing passage remains open, which it should unless the patient vomits. Remember, the convulsion will pass — it is just a big twitching of the muscles.

In a cancer patient, the symptoms of uremic poisoning almost always indicate that the end is approaching. It is just a matter of time until he or she begins sleeping deeper and longer, sometimes with one or both eyes partially open. This is a comatose state. Anything anyone wants to say to the patient better be said soon because the patient will be awake less and less.

Burst of Energy

A few days before death it is not unusual for patients to have a sudden burst of energy. Sometimes it takes the form of extreme restlessness. The patient cannot get comfortable. The bed has to be moved up and down many many times. The patient demands to be moved, but the new position is comfortable for only a minute or two and then the patient wants another position. Sometimes along with the restlessness the patient will exhibit irritability.

If the patient becomes hard to handle, there are a couple of alternatives you can try. One is to keep two or more people around the bed at all times so together you can restrain the patient. You can try speaking firmly to the patient, but this does not always work. There are soft restraints called Posey restraints, which can be used to tie the patient to the bed. Also, pain medication can be injected to sedate the patient.

The bout of energy brings on a new period where the patient drastically uses up all remaining body reserves. Bodily movements generate a lot of waste which, if accompanied by renal insufficiency, increases the overall toxicity of the body.

Typically, of the patients who experience burst of energy, it does not happen right at the end but a few days or a week before death. Some patients, particularly older patients or those in a coma, may never have an excitable period. They seem just to slip further and further into the deep quiet.

During the couple of frenetic days of activity, some family members may unrealistically be filled with hope for recovery because the patient looks like he or she is making a comeback. Suddenly, after a quiet period, perhaps the first in days, the patient will appear dramatically wasted away. The energy is gone, the body is shrinking, and the patient slips away, closer and closer to coma.

Breathing

Breathing is an important bodily function, that reflects the progress of the cancer.

There is a breathing pattern called "Cheyne-Stokes," which may occur a few days before death. You will notice that the patient pauses for long periods, ten to thirty seconds, between breaths. You will find yourself waiting at the edge of your chair for the patient to take the next breath. You think the patient has died; you sometimes hope the patient has died because it would be so easy. Then two quick breaths come. This uneven pattern usually takes place while the patient is sleeping because when awake, he monitors his breathing pattern consciously.

Another breathing problem is wheezing. If the patient was coughing and spitting up phlegm from his lungs, chances are the condition will worsen. The patient may become too weak to spit up the mucus. Each breath rattles. Eventually, the wheezing will become so loud that the heart cannot be heard with a stethoscope. General poor circulation will also result in an increased liquid content of the lungs. When the wheezing becomes very loud and the patient is too weak to spit up mucus, only a couple of days remain.

There is another breathing pattern called the "death rattle," which is loud breathing from the throat area and not from phlegm in the chest. Nurses in the hospital believe that when they hear the rattle, death is close at hand.

Coma

A coma is a deep sleep. If the comatose patient is left alone, he or she will usually slip off into a quiet death. If the patient is in a hospital where regulations dictate the use of life-supporting devices at all times, the comatose patient can live on for months aided by fluids and nutrients provided by the IV.

One important reason for dying at home is that you can do without life-supporting devices. This lets the process of dying follow its natural course if you choose. Death by coma is pleasant, as far as we know. The patient virtually goes to sleep and does not wake up. This will eventually happen even in an intensive care unit, only the end will be delayed. However, in the meantime there can be convulsions when the kidneys fail as they are prone to do eventually, and there is the human toll of keeping vigil next to a comatose body for weeks and weeks.

Cost is another consideration. Hospital care is expensive. Patients I surveyed kept insisting that the family not spend a life time's worth of savings on care that can never cure.

After Danny accepted his terminal illness, he became almost miserly with the doctor and the hospital. "My wife and kids need this money," he told me. "Why should I spend over $100 a day to be somewhere I don't want to be! And my youngest kids aren't even allowed on the ward. No way am I staying in a hospital."

In a comatose state, the patient is in a very deep sleep. We do not know for sure how much the patient registers. Most patients seem to hear and understand what we said around them even when they are semi-comatose. It is said that hearing is the last sense to go, so say only what you do not mind the patient hearing even when he or she is in a coma. The comatose patient may understand far more than we think, so continue to talk to the patient and believe that he is still aware. Touch his or her hands. Turn the patient over and give him a backrub. When you talk, tell the patient that he is loved and that you release him — he has your permission to go whenever it is time. Say you will always hold his memory close to your heart and he will live through you. Keep repeating over and over that it is all right for him or her to go, to go with love. The patient may be waiting for your release.

One family I worked with had a teenage son, Jason, who was not adjusting to his mother's illness from breast cancer. He experienced a lot of anger and depression. When his mother was comatose, Jason finally resolved his conflict and came to his mother's side, telling her that he had worked it through and he would be all right. When he finished telling her of his life plans, she patted his hand and died as though she had been waiting for Jason to release her. Once she knew he could cope, she left in peace.

An attractive woman who was dying of breast cancer loved belly dancing music. Her sister Louise played it for Susan even though the attending nurse seemed to resent it. Susan's breathing seemed to settle down when she heard the music she enjoyed or the voice of her loving sister. Louise held Susan's hand even though she had been in coma for a couple of days. Louise spoke lovingly to her of good times past. She also told Susan to feel free to go when she was ready. Susan had made all of her own arrangements to die at home, including the hiring of her own nurses. Financially comfortable, Susan wanted to remain at home but did not want to burden her family. She went fast, going from walking at the supermarket to comatose in less than a month. Susan accepted her own death and arranged matters with the grace she used throughout her life.

Typically, patients take in and feel more than they can tell us about. Continue the morphine or pain medication on regular intervals even though the patient is comatose. Since we do not know for sure, there is a chance the patient may still be feeling pain but not able to tell us.

The Final Days

Saturday

In the previous six months, Dad had been bedridden at home and occasionally in the hospital for short stays. Eleven days before he died, Dad went to the hospital again where he remained for five days, his longest stay. The obstruction in his small intestine was complete. He could eat nothing solid because there was nowhere for food to go. The only nourishment he received was from an IV. The sole output was occasional urine. He expressed very little interest in food but was thirsty from time to time. He slept in short stretches and was not awake very long. Dad was completely lucid, although he seemed to have little to say. He followed our conversations and made appropriate remarks and laughed at funny comments. With the nurses and with us, he was the perfect gentleman, considerate and compliant. He was neither depressed nor overtly angry; he just looked increasingly weak.

The entire family was at the hospital, and someone was with him all night. He became restless and had pain when we spoke about some of us going home for awhile, so we learned to slip in and out of his room without announcement. Mother was the only person whose absence really upset him, so she stayed on without leaving. The nurses brought her a rollaway, which they set up in Dad's private room so Mother could rest.

Saturday Dad became upset and depressed. He said he knew he would never get out of the hospital alive, and he wanted to be at home. He was afraid to die among strangers, he said. I promised him I would take him home as soon as possible and began making arrangements. He had never spoken so openly before about his death.

The arrangements included informing the hospital of our intention to take him home. We requested all the necessary drugs and some instruction in how to administer them and how to care for Dad, in general. We also needed to rent a hospital bed and a nasal-gastric pump.

Dad was as excited as a child at the prospect of going home. He seemed to gain new energy and interest in his surrroundings. He kept telling us that he was ready to leave the hospital.

Saturday night he slept in short stretches. His statements were not always lucid. The statements were correct grammatically but did not relate to something the listener was clued into. Some of our conversations went as follows:

"What was his name?"

"I do not know, Dad. What do you think his name was?"

"I am pretty sure it was Rick Stone."

"That is a nice strong name."

"Yes, it is."

I did not carry on the nonlucid conversation too long, just long enough to let him know someone who cared was listening. It is a boost to the patient's integrity to treat his conversation with respect rather than confront him or her with the terrible realization that they are not making sense.

Mother had a difficult time dealing with Dad's nonlucid times She feared most that his mind would go. I thought the nonlucidity was a function of the medication and the night. During the day he was lucid and delightful to talk to. His main problem during the day was figuring out the time. Only a small window in the hospital indicated whether it was day or night. His sense of time was going. Most of us can feel internally if a lot of time or a short amount of time has passed. Dad knew he could no longer judge passage of time, and this bothered him. Each time he asked what time it was, we told him the time followed by the appropriate word: morning, afternoon, evening, or night. We never said; five minutes after the last time you asked, although that was often true. We tried placing a big clock on the wall by the foot of his bed, but his eyesight was affected by the medication, and he could not make it out.

Sunday

The family now camped at the hospital around the clock. It looked as though Dad could die any moment. We brought in a coffee pot and a crock pot of soup with the hospital's permission to make ourselves comfortable. Sunday was our day for demonstrating the medical skills we were learning. Saturday we observed carefully what the nurses did. Sunday the nurses observed us as we practiced. We gave all the shots. We took turns deciding where to give the shot, loading the Tubex and inserting the needle. We changed the nasal-gastric pump when the holding jar got full, measuring its contents and recording the measure on the chart.

Dad became restless on Sunday, and he had more energy than before. He was uncomfortable but not in pain. We moved the position on his motorized hospital bed thirty-two times in one hour. He required someone constantly working on him — wiping his brow, holding an emesis bowl so he could cough and spit into it, giving him drinks of juice or feeding him sherbet.

His desire to go home was strong. We were all impatient for the doctor to sign us out. We worked hard on the diversionary techniques to keep Dad settled down. This was a very active day for all of us.

Sunday Dad talked quite a bit about dying. He said that he had accepted his death, wanted the rest of us to accept it also, and release him when the time came. He spoke about how each of his children had turned out well, doing something we could be proud of. He seemed to be summing up his life and taking stock. This was the last day that he was really verbally fluent.

Monday

When the doctor arrived early Monday, he asked Dad how he could help. Dad replied that there were two ways the doctor could help. One was to let him go home. The second was to let him die. He said he did not want to fight the death any longer.

The doctor said he respected my fahter's decisions and agreed with him. He suggested the IV be disconnected as Dad left the hospital. The N-G would be left in place because it did not prolong life, just make Dad comfortable. He promised an adequate supply of morphine, a nurse to visit us at home to help make the transition. The doctor said he enjoyed working with my father and his family. The two men shook hands as friends and the doctor left.

When we left the hospital with supplies in hand, I felt we were bursting loose from bondage, even though the hospital staff had been very accomodating. Once we got Dad at home, my good feelings changed to feelings of trepidation. I wondered what we had gotten ourselves into. Now all the responsibility for his care fell onto our shoulders. Our only backup was the doctor's nurse, who promised a house visit if something came up that we could not handle. What seemed so easy in the hospital now seemed very frightening.

We reassured each other. Karey and George made Dad's room tidy. Bonnie bustled around making Dad comfortable. I fiddled with the N-G. If this is What Dad wants, we said, it is our duty to do it. The hospital would not do any more for him.

Our fears were not quelled when we discovered that the nasal-gastric pump that had been delivered was the wrong kind. Dad needed a certain strength that worked intermittently off and on, so as not to put too much suction on his stomach. The hospital supply company delivered one that worked at a strong, steady suction. I called them and they promised to send out a messenger with a replacement, but due to the snowstorm and low temperatures, she probably would not arrive for some hours. The staff at the hospital equipment supply company also gave us instructions regarding how to make the pump we had work until they could replace it.

Karey and I worked together turning the pump on then off in twenty minute periods. We felt uncomfortable about having to improvise, but Dad did not mind. He was ecstatic about being at home. He smiled constantly.

Monday afternoon Dad rested and woke up full of energy. In the hospital he could not even roll over. Now at home, he bounced out of bed. At first we tried to restrain him. But since standing up seemed to be so important to him, we let him try standing with two people at his side in case he faltered. He seemed unsteady, but very, very proud of himself. Next to his bed was his bureau with a full length mirror. He stood in front of it, looked at himself and straightened his hair.

Dad was experiencing a burst of energy. He smiled, he sat up, he leaped out of bed. We found ourselves giving him morphine to keep him manageable. His energetic period was a time of great happiness for us, even though it was a lot of work, also. Everytime one of his grandchildren visited, Dad would hop out of bed and show that he could still stand. He laughed and played with them, clearly enjoying the youngsters who could not visit him in the hospital. His new strength did not mix well with the times when he was not lucid. Once he was talking about it being time to go to work, and he leaped out of bed. I hung on to the N-G tube so it would not pull out of his nose. Then I stood in front of him and firmly told him to return to bed. Unsteady that he was, he sat down but missed the bed. Down he went on the floor. I summoned Karey's husband George, who unselfishly did a great deal of work for us as did Bonnie's husband, Ken. George and I helped Dad get back into bed. Luckily no damage was done. Dad appeared to remember this incident, and he did not try to leave the side of the bed again without assistance.

Tuesday

Dad's activity continued all day Tuesday. He looked about the same as he did in the hospital except that he had virtually no discomfort. We gave morphine shots largely to control his restlessness and activity. We expected Dad to run a fever, since his kidneys were not working well, but he never did. He never stopped producing urine; however, it was progressively turning darker and malodorous.

He continued to understand what was going on around him. He did not speak much but he nodded at appropriate times. His activity diminished. He still sat up but only occasionally did he stand. More and more assistance was needed to move him around.

Dad's mood the entire time he was home was happy and content. When he first arrived back home from the hospital he was jubilant. Tuesday evening he began to run out of steam. He turned farther inward, but he was not depressed.

Tuesday night the first night nurse relieved us. We decided one of us would stay up with her in case Dad began jumping out of bed even though we were all pretty worn out. However, her gentle and competent manner conveyed enough trust that we left her in charge. Dad was sleeping deeply, had not stirred in three hours, and looked like he would rest through the night. We left orders to be called if his condition changed.

Wednesday

When we awoke six hours later and looked in on Dad, what we saw shocked us. Dad's frame shrank during the night. For the previous forty-eight hours he had been off all liquids, and it finally showed. His bones were visible through his skin, which seemed yellow. His breathing developed a wheeze.

Wednesday was depressing. I think during his active period, we began to harbor the unrealistic expectation that he might live a long time or even recover. We sat down together and shared our thoughts on this matter and worked out our feelings.

Wednesday was a long day mainly because there was little to do for Dad. While he requested many things Monday and Tuesday, Wednesday he lay very still and asked for nothing.

The N-G was taking out the same amount of stomach fluids this day as before. The color had gone from amber to dark brown flecks. The red blood I saw in the hospital never returned.

During the day his wheezing became louder. He only had one lung; the other was removed seventeen years previously because of cancer. It looked as though the difficulty of breathing was wearing him out.

Karey developed the habit of saying, "We know you are there behind the morphine, Dad." He seemed to be practically unconscious most of the time. He would appear to be sleeping and then his eyes would open a crack. He would stare out of his half-open eyes, apparently asleep. Sometimes his eyes would roll back and only the whites would show. Once he woke up when the morphine wore off and he said, "I am glad you know I can hear you but I can't talk." The other thing he said from time to time was "Love you."

Wednesday night we had a different night nurse. Sandy was excellent: professional and caring. She listened to Dad's lung with her stethoscope, took his blood pressure, which was normal, and checked our shot records. She pleasantly talked with anyone who remained in Dad's room and encouraged us to do as much for him as we wanted.

We went to bed around midnight, but I got up shortly afterwards because I did not like the sound of Dad's breathing, which was labored and very loud. Sandy could not hear his heart through the rattling.

Thursday

During the next two hours Dad mostly rested. I continued to rub his arm and hand and sometimes his chest. I spoke softly to him telling him how we loved him, that he was not alone, and that it was all right for him to leave when he wanted.

About four-thirty in the morning he woke up. I gave him some water. He signaled for something and looked around the room. He was holding my hand and he pulled it to his lips and kissed me. Again I told him how I loved him and how I knew he would always be with me in my thoughts. He smiled and put his head back on the pillow. He took a long, slow deep breath, and then paused. Sandy jumped up and put the stethoscope to his chest. I knocked on the wall for the family to join us. I said, "Good bye, Dad, I love you," and he took another breath. The family joined us, and he exhaled his final breath.

We stayed close to Dad after he died. Always considerate of our needs, George and Sandy stayed outside the bedroom and gave Mother and us kids a chance to be with Dad. We cried and continued to hold his hand, but no one felt that crushing, screaming anguish some people feel at a death. We saw to it that his final days were as comfortable and loving as possible.

We felt a mixture of sadness and relief. We had done all we could, and this provided us with a sense of peace and tranquility, but at the same time we were sorry Dad had to leave us. Even in his diminished capacity we enjoyed having him around. I was glad that he did not suffer. His discomfort the last two weeks was minimal and manageable. He had the most pain during his angry and depressed phases when he seemed to be fighting everyone, including his own body. Dad died a happy man, and at the time of his death he was at home surrounded by us all.

Family members contributed in slightly different ways. Of the three sons-in-law, Ken and David took care of little children and ran errands. The two sons, Mike and Tom, also ran errands and continued to go to work. They found it hard to provide hands-on comfort and care. Tom would sit in the room next to Dad for hours without speaking. Dad seemed to like the quiet since that epitomized the quiet strength he and Tom shared. The other son-in-law, George, was able to rub Dad down and speak comfortingly to him.

Of the daughters, Bonnie had been providing support over the last months. Until the last two days of Dad's life, she went to work each day and cared for her three young children, still finding a couple of hours for Dad. Karey and I remained with Dad and Mother at their home his last week plus some time after his death. Since David was caring for our boys and Karey was expecting her first child, we were able to devote ourselves round the clock to Dad. JoAnn, the college student who had recently moved out of the house, came over when she could. I think she felt a little pushed out by the rest of us and had a difficult time finding her niche. Mother was constantly available to Dad and to the rest of us as she always had been. Everyone had a chance to say what they wanted or had to say. JoAnn, perhaps, was left with some unfinished business with Dad.

As a man content with his fate, Dad was able to return our love. While we were giving a lot to him in terms of care and affection, we were getting a lot back and felt very fulfilled about the way we spent those last days. All of us unanimously agreed that if we had to do it all over again, we would do it exactly the same way, except perhaps to bring him home earlier from the hospital.

THE LIVING WILL

A living will is a quasi-legal document a person writes and signs to make provisions for the kind of medical decisions to be made on his behalf should he be unable to make his wishes known due to illness. Often a living will is composed when a person still feels healthy but is aware of a progressive illness. In the will, the person states the plans he has made and wants carried out when it comes to prolongation of his life.

Usually a living will is used by a patient with a terminal illness to specify that no extraordinary measures may be taken to keep him alive. This means no respirators or other life-supporting devices should be attached to a body that could no longer remain alive on its own. In the event the sick person is no longer able to make medical decisions, the power to make those decisions may be turned over to someone the ill person trusts.

Many healthy persons are routinely signing such documents just in case an accident might turn them into a Karen Quinlan. The life-supporting devices are capable of doing almost all of the bodily functions except return brain activity to a dead brain. Patients with no brain activity, as manifested by a flat EEG, and artificially kept alive, stay in deep coma. Muscles atrophy and the body may pull itself into a fetal position.

To the cancer patient the thought of living without the ability to be in charge of one's own body is frightening. Turning over this decision-making power to a trusted person who knows what the patient wants relieves much tension. A living will ensures that a family member can come home for care even though the patient may be unable to sign himself out of the hospital. The will gives the family the power to sign the patient out to go home.

Living wills can specify organ donation or turning over part of the body to the local medical school so perhaps something can be learned about the progress of this kind of cancer.

I believe a patient should be kept by whatever medical methods it takes for as long as the patient wishes to live. Some patients will choose to live for a long time under greatly reduced capacity. The ability to let go and say "Enough of this kind of life!" is not a one-time choice made when healthy. It is a long process whereby the patient thinks about it for days, pondering his condition. The decision is difficult because some days are better than others and things might look improved for awhile. Finally, the overall downhill pattern is all too obvious.

When a patient says he has had enough and wants to let go, reconsider this decision for several days. You can tell that the patient is sure about the appropriateness of this decision by the conviction in the voice and the adamant refusal of food, liquid, or any more drugs except pain killers. When the final decision is reached, the patient should be helped to go with love. Tell him or her that it is all right to leave.

The Natural Death Act (1976) in California recognizes the right of adults to prepare living wills. They may contain written instructions authorizing their doctors to withhold or withdraw life-sustaining procedures in the specified conditions of terminal illness or irreversible accidents.

Other states are following with their own legislation. Minnesota, for instance, recognizes the right of people to set up "conservatorships." Here a healthy person can turn over his right to make his own medical decisions to a trusted loved one who has in writing the guidelines for what the patient wants. This right is automatically transferred if the patient is too incapacitated to make his own choices.

One of the major reasons for legislative action is to relieve doctors and hospitals from being sued by family members for carrying out the patient's directives for being allowed to die naturally. The law also states that choosing natural death with dignity does not constitute suicide, so insurance companies cannot withhold payment for that reason.

Since each state varies in how they stand regarding living wills, it is not a bad idea to contact a lawyer if you want to be sure that your document will be honored. Otherwise, you can use the living wills provided here either as written or with whatever modifications you want to make. Notarize the version you want and send a copy to your doctor. See what he says. Ask how he feels about cutting off life-sustaining equipment and procedures when there is not hope. In my experience, most doctors are in agreement with stopping extraordinary measures when all reasonable hope for recovery is gone.

To my family, my physician, my lawyer, and my clergyman:

If the time comes when I can no longer take part in decisions for my own future, let this statement stand as the testament of my wishes:

If there is no reasonable expectation of my recovery from physical or mental disability, I —, request that I be allowed to die and not to be kept alive by artificial or heroic measures. Death is as much a reality as birth, growth, maturity, and old age. I believe it is the one certainty I cannot escape. I do not fear death as much as I fear the indignity of deterioration and being surrounded by strangers in this final phase of my life. I respectfully request that I remain at home cared for by the people I have lived my life with. I ask them to continue to administer pain-killing drugs to me even if they hasten the moment of death. However, I do not want my life prolonged by the use of any equipment such as mechanical ventilators, intensive care services, antibiotics, or blood products.

This request is made after careful consideration. Although this document may not be legally binding, you who care for me will, I hope, feel morally bound to follow its mandate. I recognize that it places a heavy burden of responsibility upon you, and it is with the intention of sharing that responsibility and of mitigating any feelings of guilt that this statement is made.

This document was prepared while I was still physically and mentally healthy. I trust it will not conflict with hospital policies. If this should happen, I request to be taken home as my first choice or taken to another hospital where my wishes can be carried out, as my second choice. I want to leave a heart-felt thanks to those family members and medical personnel who cooperate in helping me die at home with dignity as I request.

Signed _____

*Witnessed by*_____

Date _____

INDEX